DICTIONARY OF PSYCHOPATHOLOGY

BY THE AUTHOR IN RELATED FIELDS

Group Psychotherapy and Personality: Intersecting Structures
Sleep Disorders: Insomnia and Narcolepsy
The Psychoanalysis of Symptoms
The Four Steps to Peace of Mind: The Simple Effective Way to Cure Our Symptoms
Love Is Not Enough: What It Takes to Make It Work

COAUTHORED BOOKS

Psychopathology and Differential Diagnosis: A Primer, with Anthony Burry
Vol. 1: *History of Psychopathology*
Vol. 2: *Diagnostic Primer*
Handbook of Psychodiagnostic Testing: Analysis of Personality in the Psychological Report, with Anthony Burry
The Emotions Profile Index, with Robert Plutchik

EDITED BOOKS

Group Cohesion: Theoretical and Clinical Perspectives
The Nightmare: Psychological and Biological Foundations

COEDITED BOOKS

Emotion: Theory, Research, and Experience, with Robert Plutchik
Vol. 1: *Theories of Emotion*
Vol. 2: *Emotions in Early Development*
Vol. 3: *Biological Foundations of Emotion*
Vol. 4: *The Measurement of Emotion*
Vol. 5: *Emotion, Psychopathology, and Psychotherapy*

DICTIONARY OF PSYCHOPATHOLOGY

Henry Kellerman

Columbia University Press New York

Columbia University Press
Publishers Since 1893
New York Chichester, West Sussex

Library of Congress Cataloging-in-Publication Data
Dictionary of psychopathology / [edited by] Henry Kellerman.
p. ; cm.
Includes bibliographical references.
ISBN 978-0-231-14650-0 (cloth : alk. paper) —
ISBN 978-0-231-14651-7 (pbk. : alk. paper)
1. Psychology, Pathological—Dictionaries. I. Kellerman, Henry.
[DNLM: 1. Psychopathology—Dictionary—English. WM 13
D55384 2009]

RC437.D53 2009
616.89003—dc22

2008031543

Casebound editions of Columbia University Press books are printed on permanent and durable acid-free paper.

Printed in the United States of America

c 10 9 8 7 6 5 4 3 2 1
p 10 9 8 7 6 5 4 3 2 1

To the memory of
Robert Plutchik
scientist, teacher,
friend, brother

CONTENTS

EDITORIAL BOARD

PREFACE

Psychopathology is ubiquitous. With respect to theory, diagnosis, and treatment, therefore, a dictionary of psychopathology is relevant to the entire cross section of mental health disciplines. This dictionary is intended to provide definitions of the concepts and vicissitudes of psychopathology as reflected within the broad theoretical domains of psychiatry, psychology, psychoanalysis, and social work as well as within the wide varieties of therapeutic modalities, such as the relational therapies, the cognitive behavioral approaches, with even a nod to the newest domain within neuroscience, that of neuropsychoanalysis—the attempt to relate brain and mind.

In keeping with this approach, this *Dictionary of Psychopathology* is shaped according to the needs of clinicians, academicians, and researchers who are professionally occupied with the subject matter of psychopathology—from psychoanalysts to behavior therapists, from ego psychologists to cognitive psychologists, from psychodynamically oriented group therapists to Gestaltists and Tavistockians, from relational therapists—including intersubjectivists, object relationists, Rogerians, and existentialists—to Jungians, from active psychotherapists to self psychologists, and from academic psychologists to neuroscientists.

Entries focus more on psychodynamic metapsychology than on cognitive behavior, a consideration based largely on the overall amplification and cumulative archive of psychodynamic psychology inspired by the expansion of interest in psychoanalysis over the span of the entire twentieth century. The ferment in psychodynamic psychology spawned a vast theoretical and clinical literature. In contrast, although cognitive behavioral approaches also go back one hundred years, its explosive history, momentum, and burgeoning theoretical and clinical literature is a more modern phenomenon. Thus the cognitive behavioral archive is a younger dimension in the unearthing of the nature of psychopathology. The relative viable age of each domain—that of psychodynamic psychology, on the one hand, and cognitive behavioral approaches, on the other—accounts for the difference in the number of entries in this dictionary that represent the two domains.

In the history of dictionary resources of psychopathology, a close examination of the literature will reveal that each of these reference works was compiled along sectarian lines: there are dictionaries for psychiatrists, most or all of which are entitled "Psychiatric Dictionary," dictionaries for psychologists, most or all of which are entitled "Dictionary of Psychology," dictionaries for psychoanalysts, most or all of which are entitled "Dictionary of Psychoanalysis," and a dictionary for social workers entitled "Dictionary of Social Work."

It is evident that extant dictionaries representing the various disciplines of the psychological sciences are characterized, parsed, and defined by their respective and particular lexicons and thus contain multitudes of entries not always, and even not always specifically, directed to the clinician, nor even, in this respect, particularly relevant to clinical concerns regarding psychopathology. For example, an entry such as *Tromner's sign,* which refers to hemiplegia (caused by organic brain disease), would probably be of little use to the clinician who is managing a private clinical practice, functioning in an agency, clinic, hospital, or psychoanalytic institute, or teaching psychopathology/abnormal psychology to undergraduates, graduates, or medical students—whether utilizing either psychodynamically oriented approaches or cognitive behavioral ones, because Tromner's sign is simply acknowledging that a snapping of the index finger will produce a flexion of the thumb. Another example would be an entry such as *hippus,* which refers to pupil contraction and dilation to light stimulation that, because of its remotest relevance to clinicians in the study of psychopathology as well as its nonexistence in the clinical psychological literature or, for that matter, in clinical practice, would also not be included.

In contrast, terms such as *projection,* defined as a defense mechanism and applied to the study of ego defenses as well as to diagnostic phenomena such as paranoia, is, of course, here registered. Another example of an entry that is included is *ego-syntonic,* because it, too, is central to clinical work with respect to the diagnostic and infrastructural understanding of anxiety and character formation, especially psychological symptom formation. A third example, the reference to the *good enough mother,* is salient to issues of psychological development and therefore also relevant to the goal and vision of this dictionary. Other examples of entries that are registered here include *systematic desensitization,* a reference to how the history of conditioning psychology has influenced the treatment of phobias, or *hot cognition,* a concept of *cognitive behavior therapy.* Even in the domain of neuropsychoanalysis, the concept of *repression of trauma* would be attributed to the phenomenon of hormone action, the result of the *retranscribing action of the hippocampus*—a region of the brain.

Thus, in view of the aim of this dictionary, it is composed and formatted in an effort to unify and encompass the true generic issue that cuts across all the mental health/scientific disciplines, sectarian lines, metapsychologies, and treatment technologies—the cohesion and synthesis of psychopathology.

In identifying psychopathology, this *Dictionary of Psychopathology* contains representation of both the wide scope of theoretical formulations as well as of the treatment technologies that correspond to these approaches. Therefore, definitions in the dictionary are guided by a fundamental tetrad of criteria:

1. that psychopathology as aberrant behavior is embedded in the personality structure—whether considered from psychoanalytic, cognitive behavioral, or relational psychologies;

2. that, in order to better appreciate psychopathological manifestations, one needs to have the opportunity to reference the parameters, fabric, and organizational nature of the entire personality network, i.e., emotion and trait development, cognitive organization, intrapsychic balance, psychosomatic correlates, diagnostic disposition, dreams and nightmares, influence of the "other," and all other vicissitudes of the personality;
3. that it is an imperative to include overall therapeutic principles and their corresponding treatment technologies in the approach to understanding both aberrant or abnormal behavior as well as normal development; and
4. that diagnosis is the code language for entire clusters of symptoms and syndromes of psychopathology.

Along with students, this dictionary will be useful to psychologists, social workers, psychiatrists, psychoanalysts, psychiatric nurses, family medical practitioners, school psychologists, counselors, and psychotherapists, as well as to other allied professionals such as academic psychologists and those with professorial positions in university undergraduate and graduate mental health programs, in medical schools, and in clinical postdoctoral institutes. Thus this dictionary is not relevant solely to one or another of the mental health disciplines. Rather, it is devoted to the specific glossary of psychopathology, relevant to all of these disciplines and to the variety of theoretical schools—to the entire arc of the mental health field.

The *Dictionary of Psychopathology* contains more than two thousand entries directed to the understanding of psychopathology, specific symptom disorders, general syndromes, various facets of the structure of personality, and diagnosis—including selected entries on the diagnostic nomenclature of the professional psychological and psychiatric associations. As such, psychological phenomena that reflect the known overall boundary of metapsychology, associated psychotherapeutic treatment technologies, and specific psychological phenomena are embraced within these entries. In addition, a wide sample of the many theoreticians and researchers, and their contributions to the understanding of psychopathology, are noted. These include representatives of the generation of pioneer contributors who formulated the necessary insights that laid the foundation for the established understanding of psychopathology and whose ideas essentially constitute benchmark advances in the history and evolution of the subject matter. Along with these seminal figures, the more contemporary theoreticians who are hewing newer insights into the understanding of psychopathology are also included and their contributions noted.

As a utilitarian repository source, this *Dictionary of Psychopathology* is designed to be easily accessed. To that end and to facilitate the unfolding of meanings, of the more than two thousand entries, over fifteen hundred are primary entries, and more than five hundred are subentries. In addition, cross-referencing is indicated throughout.

The editorial board of this dictionary reviewed definitions of entries embracing the broad prism of psychopathology including psychodynamic/psychoanalytic, relational, cognitive behavioral, and other psychological therapies, also covering theoretical formulations that characterize a variety of phenomena of the psychiatric and psychological literatures. In addition, conceptualization of differential diagnosis specifically and psychodiagnostics generally was considered as well as references to psychopharmacological listings and the relation of neuroscience to psychological phenomena.

To underscore the promise of this dictionary, it is hoped that its mission has been reasonably approximated—to address psychopathology from a synthesizing point of advantage—so that parameters of personality, character formation, derived psychopathology such as symptoms, treatment concepts, and diagnoses, are identified and cogently defined. In this way psychopathology, as the essential substance of the dictionary, is surrounded by the panorama of metapsychologies and the sweep of therapeutic modalities.

This comprehensive approach to the analysis of psychopathology also implies that the terminology of this dictionary does not solely reflect the problems of clinical patients. We need to remember, as already stated, that psychopathology is ubiquitous.

DICTIONARY OF PSYCHOPATHOLOGY

A

ABANDONMENT REACTION Catastrophic emotional reaction to loss as in a sense of severe deprivation, loneliness, and depression, along with feelings of alienation, helplessness, or disempowerment, accompanied consciously by tension and fear and, perhaps unconsciously and more profoundly, by suppressed anger.

ABCDE Albert Ellis formulated the ABCDE model to facilitate client's utilization of REBT (rational emotive behavior therapy) as a self-help method.

A stands for "activating event." This event can be past, present, or anticipated.

B stands for "beliefs" about the activating event. IBs are irrational beliefs, RBs are rational and reality based.

C stands for "consequences." Irrational beliefs lead to dysfunctional emotional and behavioral consequences; rational beliefs to more adaptive feelings and behaviors.

D stands for "disputing" irrational beliefs. This is done through client's asking themselves questions such as how are these thoughts helping me feel better and do better? Where's the evidence that this belief is true? Is this situation really awful and intolerable?

E stands for "effective" new philosophies / beliefs that result from disputing IBs. Such beliefs are characterized by preferences rather than demands, seeing things as hassles rather than horrors, and evaluating people's behavior rather than their entire worth.

ABERRANT BEHAVIOR Referring to maladaptive, or maladjusted behavior, or behavior that deviates from normal or expected responses. Divergence from the normal needs to be an obvious skewed behavior that reflects a significant severity of disturbance.

ABNORMAL PSYCHOLOGY The study of mental and emotional disorders as well as aberrant behavior. In clinical discourse, abnormal psychology is also referred to as psychopathology.

ABREACTION Discharge of emotion from a repressed state. Usually seen as connecting the emotion to a forgotten memory and, as a result, is defined as the basis of a catharsis—of feeling better.

ABSTRACTING DISABILITY Inability to analogize or in other ways utilize abstraction from concrete information.

ACAROPHOBIA Fear of skin infestation by crawling organisms. See Phobia.

ACCIDENT PRONENESS In classical psychoanalytic understanding, frequent accidents implies a strong superego so that the person punishes the self because of the alleged presence of unconscious anger and guilt.

ACCULTURATED NEED Part of the adaptational theory proposed by Rado. See Need.

ACE TEST An intelligence test for high school students or older, designed by the American Council on Education.

ACROPHOBIA Fear of heights. See Phobia.

ACTING IN The acting in concept was developed to identify repressive phenomena within the psychotherapeutic session, with respect to repression of feelings toward the therapist. Hypothetically, the repression would be of anger. Thus acting in is not a matter of injudicious behavior of an acting out episode.

ACTING OUT The psychiatric definition is centered on behavior considered delinquent, inappropriate, or age inappropriate. In contrast, the psychoanalytic definition connects behavior with repression, thus revealing a psychological dynamic to the acting out. As such, acting out is considered "doing instead of knowing." Acting out, therefore, becomes the unconscious attempt not to know something, not to have insight about the "something" or to remain unconscious regarding the meaning of the "something." Instead the person does something motorically, that is, behaviorally and repetitively. In this sense acting out is a replacement for the memory of something and someone and thus becomes the neurotic translation of memory into behavior. Hypothetically, acting out (in order not to know something) is an attempt to repress anger. In its historical context the repressed anger (or rage) is directed toward a specific person and then becomes displayed in the present through injudicious behavior. Such anger as represented by the acting out is considered to be a basic transferential reaction to a historic parental figure. Thus the continual discharge of tension in the acting out behavior can be understood as a repetitive attempt to master the original drive demand for expression of the anger as it connects with the memory of the original historic figure or current transferential figure. To trace the psychological vicissitudes of acting out would be equivalent to unfolding the entire template of psychoanalytic metapsychology, because what would be revealed would include everything from defense mechanisms represented by repression, to the structure of the unconscious, to drive demand, to the appearance of psychological-emotional symptoms, to transference, to repetition compulsion, and to the psychology of resistance in treatment.

ACTIVE THERAPY A confrontational system of therapy developed by Stekel. Influenced also by the experiential encounter movement of the 1960s exemplified by the work of William Shutz.

ACTIVITY GROUP THERAPY Slavson's formulation to facilitate the emotional growth of children who are particularly shy or experiencing difficulty in social interaction by exposing them to supportive social groups. These groups can go on trips or otherwise plan activities together. See Slavson.

ACULALIA Speech that sounds both to the subject as well as to others like gibberish—usually a result of receptive and / or expressive aphasia. See Aphasia.

ACUTE BRAIN DISORDER Sometimes referred to as an organic brain disorder or even organic psychosis. Caused by brain trauma and, because of its acute nature, is frequently reversible. Such persons will usually show poor frustration tolerance and as a result will behave impulsively and can have temper outbursts.

ACUTE SCHIZOPHRENIA See Schizophrenia.

ADAPTATION Generally considered important in the development of socially mature behavior. Freud's adaptive theory examines the relation of ego to the environment with a focus on reality testing and secondary process. See Freud; reality testing; secondary process.

ADAPTATION SYNDROME, GENERAL See general adaptation syndrome.

ADAPTATIONAL PSYCHODYNAMICS From Rado. Essentially a psychoanalytic system that examines levels of adaptation within the broad framework of motivation and impulse / control issues.

ADLER, ALFRED (1870–1937). European psychiatrist who focused on inferiority feelings, compensatory defense, and a superiority syndrome, and ultimately identified his orientation as individual psychology. Adler, unlike Freud, postulated only a single drive that motivates all personality and behavior. While Freud focused on the past, Adler looked to the future insofar as he felt that goals drive people: that is to say, a person is teleologically programmed—always aiming toward the goal. He developed a system of understanding the relationship of birth order to personality and formulated what he called the three dominant desires (motivations).

The getting desire—this is an oral-type person who is vulnerable to dependency problems and depression;

The avoiding desire—this is a person who remains detached;

The socially useful desire—this is a person who is able to share.

Adler also conceived of a typology based on his system that included three basic types plus one other:

The avoiding type—can become psychotic under stress;
The leaning type—dependent and can develop phobias, obsessions, anxiety, hysteria;
The ruling type—dominant and not terribly empathetic;
The socially useful type—healthy.

Other vicissitudes of "will" for Adler included

will to be above—the woman's need to be like the man, understood in psychoanalytic theory to be a function of a compensatory need;
will to be up—striving for a more obvious presentation of masculine aggression;
will to power—the person will do most anything to avoid a feminine identification, rather striving toward a definitive masculine identification

AFFECT This term is frequently used interchangeably with that of emotion. It has also been understood as a quanta of energy that is attached to ideas or as easily to objects—that is, people. The psychic mechanism of displacement, for example, acts to make flexible the potential of affect to attach to a variety of objects (people) so that the true "who" toward whom the affect was originally intended can be hidden or concealed—especially from the self. Such displacement is a component of a repression cluster of defenses. Other synonyms for affect include mood, and feeling. Affect can also refer to the extent to which a person's emotions are generally palpable. Mood can refer to the state of the person's optimism or pessimism. Feeling can refer to one's empathy index. In neuropsychoanalysis, affects are considered to be generated in response to emotion-provoking stimuli in the right limbic system (amygdale anterior cingulated, orbitofrontal cortex) and autonomic nervous system.

AFFECT CONTAGION Originating in the work of Sullivan, this concept presaged intersubjectivity theory's emphasis on the context sensitivity of affect.

AFFECT DISTURBANCE One of Bleuler's four factors of diagnosis for schizophrenia. The other factors are ambivalence, associative disturbance, and autism. These are called the four *A*s. Affect disturbance elements include flat or blunted affect and / or lability of affect or inappropriate affect.

AFFECT DYSREGULATION In neuropsychoanalysis, short-term affect dysregulation expressed as an anger dyscontrol may be characterized by reduced serotonergic activity.

AFFECT HUNGER Desperation for affection seen in rejected children.

AFFECT REGULATION In cognitive behavior therapy, the use of strategies such as cognitive restructuring or relaxation to alter an emotional state.

AFFECTIVE DISORDERS Disturbances of mood as in manic / depressed. In the *Diagnostic and Statistical Manual* of the American Psychiatric Association, affective disorders are listed as mood disorders. For the most part they include mood episodes, depressive disorders, and bipolar disorders.

AFFECTIVE PROCEDURAL MEMORY See Transmuting internalization.

AFFECTIVE TRANSFORMATION The phenomenon by which emotionally charged values tend to expand and increase in all respects.

AFFINITY HYPOTHESIS See Antagonism hypothesis.

AGCT (ARMY GENERAL CLASSIFICATION TEST) An intelligence test used for people who have had formal education.

AGGRESSION An attempt to gain the ascendancy through attacking behavior or implemented anger or force that can also include emotions of fury and rage. Related, but not inextricably, to hate or hostility. Can be directed simply to achieve a goal, yet usually refers to a destructive drive. Is antithetical to libido and should be distinctly contrasted with assertion, which is not necessarily aggressive. In Freudian psychology, aggression is a derivative of the death instinct. See Anger; Serotonin.

AGITATED DEPRESSION Depression with anxiety, irritability, and impatience.

AGNOSIA Disturbance of language with respect to the recognition of symbols.

Orientation agnosia—In neuropsychoanalytic investigations within the domain of neuroscience, this is a visuospatial cognition regarding object recognition where the subject may understand an object but be unable to relate to it in its proper spatial axis.

AGORAPHOBIA Fear of open spaces. The natural deterioration of functioning in such a person can be illustrated by a progression in which the person at first cannot leave the building to go to work, then cannot leave the apartment itself, then cannot leave the bedroom, and, finally, drawing the circumference and parameter of life to an even more confined space, cannot leave the bed.

AIM INHIBITION Describes, in psychoanalysis, an absence of libidinal interest in another, as in a platonic relationship.

ALARM REACTION Clinically considered to be a reaction to the stance of vigilance seen in anxiety and / or paranoid conditions; it is also seen as part of the general adaptation syndrome. See General adaptation syndrome.

ALEXANDER, F. MATTHIAS (1869–1955). See Alexander Technique.

ALEXANDER, FRANZ (1891–1964). European psychoanalyst known for his theory of psychosomatic disorders. Alexander promoted the idea of verbal encoragement in therapy in contrast to the so-called blank screen classical analytic stance.

ALEXANDER TECHNIQUE A therapy to address repetitive habits, thinking, and muscular tension devised by Matthias F. Alexander, an Australian Shakespearean actor. Through a hands-on mind-body approach, the aim of the therapy is to help the subject better calibrate a kinesthetic and postural sense aimed at reducing stress.

ALEXITHYMIA Inability to understand feelings so that communicating ideas and / or affect is not well accomplished. Also associated with autism.

ALIENATION Estrangement from interpersonal relationships and even from the self or parts of the self.

ALL OR NONE REACTION The observation that instinctive reactions, usually in the form of motor responses, occur completely or not at all.

ALLOPLASTY Managing the environment by changing it. Contrasts with autoplasty—managing difficulty by changing the self. See Autoplasty.

ALLPORT, GORDON W. (1897–1967). American psychologist who underscored the importance of focusing on personality traits and developed the influential trait theory of personality.

ALTER EGO TRANSFERENCE See Transference.

ALZHEIMER'S DISEASE A form of dementia occurring later in life and ending in death within five to ten years of onset.

AMBIVALENCE Opposite emotions or wishes pulling in opposite directions: a *yes* versus a *no.* The problem is that ambivalence is not democratic—the *yes* gets a single vote, whereas the *no* gets two. Especially emphasized in obsessional states. It is one of Bleuler's four *A*s, used as criteria for diagnosing schizophrenia, although by itself it is certainly not pathognomonic of psychosis. Considered by some to be the coexistence of love and hate. Stranger anxiety is seen as the beginning of ambivalence in the child. See Schizophrenia.

AMBULATORY SCHIZOPHRENIA See Schizophrenia.

AMNESIA Loss of memory.

Retrograde amnesia is loss of memory even before the onset of the traumatic event. See Psychogenic amnesia.

Anterogradeamnesia is a loss of memory regarding events occurring post trauma.

AMPHETAMINES "Uppers" or "speed": energizers frequently used to treat ADHD children. Seen as a paradoxical reaction; that is, use of an energizer to calm an overenergetic child.

AMYGDALA A brain organ associated with the memory of emotional events and implicated in the expression of aggression.

ANACLITIC Referring to the nature of bonding. Narcissistic choices are based on a choice of someone resembling the self, while anaclitic choices reflect similarity of the object to the childhood dependency figure such as the mother or other primary caregiver.

ANACLITIC DEPRESSION Coined by René Spitz (1887–1974), European psychoanalyst. Refers to the three-month age of the child when separated from the mother. After such separation the infant demonstrates a lack of interest in the environment accompanied by a pronounced listlessness, poor appetite, and fitful sleep. It has been reported that the anaclitic state subsides if the mother returns. If the infant's relationship with the mother before separation was bad, as in the "bad mother," the anaclitic depression does not ignite. Only if the mother was a "good mother," will the anaclitic depression appear after separation: loss is only meaningful if the relationship was good. The corollary is that loss, as descriptive of a bad relationship, reflects arithmetic subtraction and is not the same as a dynamic emotional reaction of loss when the relationship was good.

ANACLITIC OBJECT Object choice defined as the difference between the subject and the object. The opposite of narcissistic object choice where libido is invested in one's own ego.

ANAL CHARACTER Personality traits derived from anal stage developmental issues include parsimony, orderliness, and compulsivity. Also related to the defense of reaction formation and the diagnosis of obsessional neurosis.

ANAL EROTICISM Libido is cathected (invested) with reference to anal stage activity and, later, to derived personality features.

ANAL RETENTION Retaining fecal matter during toilet training and theoretically assumed to correlate to the appearance of future personality traits such as stubbornness.

ANAL SADISM Gratification from the infliction of pain or cruel behavior on another.

ANAL STAGE Pleasure fixations organized during the anal stage of development. Part of Freud's psychosexual stages of development: oral, anal, phallic, oedipal.

ANAL TRIAD Three main traits of the anal personality or character structure are orderliness, obstinacy, and parsimony.

ANALYSAND The patient. Refers to the psychoanalytic student who is in the process of a "training analysis"—the self in psychoanalysis.

ANALYTICAL THERAPY Referring to Jung's approach in which compensatory mechanisms are brought to bear on the conflict between conscious and unconscious material. The objective is for consciousness to prevail. See Jung, Carl.

ANAMNESTIC DATA Detailed investigation of patient's history.

ANCHORING SYMPTOMS Those symptoms that are pathognomonic or central to any diagnosis. Developed by psychiatrist Otto Kernberg, who studied borderline and narcissistic pathology. See Kernberg, Otto.

ANESTHESIA, GLOVE Thought to be a hysterical reaction insofar as the person cannot feel or sense the bare hand or hand covered by a glove.

ANGER Arguably the most frequently experienced emotion based upon the observation that we are all wish-soaked creatures and that the wishes people have are most frequently thwarted, denied, or postponed because it is not possible to control all of life's variables, which impinge upon any given wish or event. Such delay to the gratification of the wish leads to feelings of disempowerment where most often the only way to become reempowered is through feeling consciously angry. The feeling of anger then constitutes a regaining of power—a reempowerment. The ubiquitousness of wishes and their frequent frustration implicates anger as the most frequently experienced of all the emotions. Anger may be construed as containing a personality—unidimensional though it is. As a basic emotion, it is tropistic insofar as it responds only to its one imperative—to expand, attack, or explode. The personality profile of anger has been proposed by Kellerman:

Anger has an aggressive drive. It's inborn.
Anger is expansive. It wants to get bigger.
Anger feels confrontational. It wants to get tough.
Anger has an entitled frame of mind. It feels it has the right to get tough.

Anger has an attack inclination. It wants to attack.
Anger wants to burst forth. It has explosive potential.
Anger sees itself as an empowerment, thereby nullifying helplessness.

A high-probability paradigm for understanding functional psychopathology concerns the likely hypothesis that suppressed anger is the implicated factor in all psychopathology so that in any deterioration of a psychopathological nature a malignant high-intensity anger such as rage (usually unconscious), radiates the personality with a force that is difficult to restrain. The accelerated downward spiral of such an inexorable eruptive and sick psychopathological deterioration, in all its morbidity, will continue to disable the afflicted person to the level of severe maladjustment and psychosis: the suppressed or repressed unconscious anger, with its attack nature, now turns on the self. This is the self attacking the self and simultaneously existing in a conscious state of disempowerment. The implication here is that in any therapeutic intervention (psychotherapy and / or medication) the target of the intervention must address the unconscious anger (as well locating its true external object)—perhaps the culprit variable in all of psychopathology. See Symptom.

ANHEDONIA Inability to experience pleasure. See Hedonism.

ANIMA Concept developed by psychiatrist Carl Jung and referring to the component of the psyche that is connected to the unconscious. The anima is in direct contrast to the persona, which is the character of the person seen by others. This is Jung's concept of soul and refers also to the unconscious female image in men, while the animus is the unconscious male image in women. All people are presumed to possess an anima and an animus in any balance, of course calibrated differently for each person.

ANIMAL METAPHORS Projective technique in which the subject chooses an animal that he would want to be like most and least, then explaining the reasons for it. Can be part of the typical projective battery of tests including the Rorschach, Thematic Apperception Test, and Machover Draw a Person Test.

ANIMUS See Anima.

ANNA O. Breuer's famous patient who had hysterical symptoms, ultimately enabling Freud, in discussions with Breuer, to theorize that such symptoms could be subject to cure through analysis.

ANNIHILATION ANXIETY See Winnicott, D. W.

ANNIVERSARY REACTION An unconscious acting out on an anniversary date, presumably as an attempt to master some previous trauma. Of course, as is the case with acting out, the original trauma is never mastered and the acting out on such an anniversary date becomes an example of Freud's repetition compulsion.

ANNIVERSARY TRANSFERENCE A person's obsessional belief that some untoward past event such as the death of a parent will be replayed years later with respect to the self and on the same anniversary date. See Anniversary reaction.

ANOREXIA NERVOSA Listed as an eating disorder in the psychiatric nosology. Usually seen in adolescent and young women obsessed with weight loss and engaged in corresponding compulsive behavior regarding loss of appetite and refusal to eat. It is hypothesized that a repressed and impacted rage toward a primary figure is the culprit in the formation of the symptom. The symptom is accompanied by the condition of amenorrhea and frequently depression. Other diagnostic references that have been correlated include obsessive, hysteric, and schizophrenic functioning. Mirror gazing and thinking "not thin enough" characterizes typical body image problems of such a person. Long periods of food deprivation occurs in the restricting type of this disorder, while binging and purging can be seen in the expansive type. Kellerman has theorized that, like all symptoms, anger is the underlying emotion here, so that gazing in the mirror and always thinking "not thin enough!" is the apparent conscious thought that replaces the actual unconscious feeling of "the anger is still there." Thus it becomes obvious that getting thinner and thinner is never going to erase the anger. Only surfacing into consciousness what exists below (the anger) and then identifying the person toward whom that anger was directed and analyzing the particular relationship can ever cure the symptom. See Symptom.

ANOSOGNOSIA In neuropsychoanalytic understanding this is a disorder of denial in which the subject, in the aftermath of a brain lesion, is unaware of some deficit of functioning. Were the deficit to be acknowledged, the anosognosia is thought to be a defense against emotional trauma. It is the maintaining of false beliefs.

ANTABUSE Pharmacological treatment for alcoholism.

ANTAGONISM HYPOTHESIS Refers to the appearance of one disorder that blocks the appearance of any second disorder. The affinity hypothesis is the opposite, insofar as it is predicted that the appearance of one disorder will increase the probability of the appearance of a second disorder.

ANTI-ANXIETY MEDICATIONS (ANXIOLYTICS) The anxiolytics include benzodiazepines, azaspirones, beta-blockers, and even antidepressants. Medications include treatment for generalized anxiety disorder, panic, phobia, obsessive-compulsive disorder, and posttraumatic stress disorder. A sampling of these medications are

benzodiazepines—such as Xanax, Valium, Ativan, Klonopin, Serax, Tranxene;
azaspirones—Buspar;
beta-blockers—Inderal, Tenormin.

See Antidepressants.

ANTICATHEXIS OR COUNTERCATHEXIS Attempt by the ego to sustain repression and control over impulses. In psychodynamic psychotherapeutic treatment a derivative mechanism crystallizes as resistance.

ANTIDEPRESSANT MEDICATIONS There are several types of antidepressants:

tricyclics—such as Elavil, Tofranil, Pamelor;
MAO Inhibitors—such as Nardil, Parnate;

selective serotonin reuptake inhibitors—such as Celexa, Lexapro, Prozac, Paxil, Zoloft;
others—Wellbutrin, Effexor, Remeron.

Antidepressants may have side effects such as changes in appetite as well as changes in fullness of libido. See Psychotropic drugs; Serotonin.

ANTIPSYCHOTIC MEDICATIONS These are labeled older typical antipsychotics and newer atypical antipsychotics.

The older typical ones include Thorazine, Haldol, Trilafon, Stelazine.
The newer atypical ones include Clozaril, Risperdal, Abilify, Seroquel, Zyprexa.

ANTISOCIAL PERSONALITY Synonymous with psychopathic or sociopathic personality. Such persons engage in varieties of acting out behaviors such as lying or stealing. Listed in the psychiatric nomenclature as a personality disorder because of the inflexible nature of the person's characteristic behavior patterns. Such difficulties are seen in the areas of cognition, emotion, interpersonal functioning, and impulse control. Difficulty in social as well as occupational arenas of functioning becomes evident.

ANXIETY A generalized tension state. Two conditions of anxiety have been delineated.

- *Automatic anxiety*—the subject is reflexively overwhelmed. Such tension is associated mostly with infants and children who are not able to integrate untoward stimuli because of an immature ego state.
- *Signal anxiety*—a term coined by Freud and applied to typical neurotic functioning; akin to Pavlovian conditioned responses by which the person anticipates dissatisfying and distasteful impending situations. The psychoanalytic conception of such anxiety (or tension) includes a developmental sequence of worry that is attached to stages of development: first, separation anxiety occurring early on before the age of two, then fear of loss of love up to two years of age, then classic

castration fears at three, and finally, as an addendum to the castration stage and an introduction to the oedipal phase, the appearance of superego derivatives of guilt and punishment.

An example of another concept of the appearance of anxiety is that developed by Kellerman, who considers anxiety to be a symptom and posits repressed anger as the source of derived tension or anxiety. Anxiety would be the radiating tension from the unconscious, implying that in the unconscious exists anger toward a particular person—a "who." This repressed unconscious anger releases tension that rises into consciousness in the form of anxiety. This is quite different from Freud's original conception of anxiety, which he first considered to be a function of repressed libidinous drive. Freud eventually relinquished this position in favor of his new conception, positing that anxiety is the function of an overwhelmed psyche unable to manage the tension from intense stimuli. In effect, psychoanalytically, anxiety is also seen as the threat of repression lifting and / or a threat to the ego. Another specific form of anxiety includes persecutory anxiety of the paranoid variety. See Signal anxiety.

ANXIETY, FREE-FLOATING Equivalent to generalized anxiety whereby no single event or person has yet been identified as the cause of the tension and disturbance.

ANXIETY, PERFORMANCE Tension associated with sexual performance, but clinical usage also refers to performance anxiety as related to that associated with any task defined as requiring a performance. For example, such anxiety can be seen in stage actors.

ANXIETY, SEPARATION See Separation anxiety.

ANXIETY, SIGNAL See Signal anxiety.

ANXIETY, STRANGER See Stranger anxiety.

ANXIETY ATTACK A severe and overwhelming sense of tension, heart palpitations, sweating, and a condensed focus on one's experience of vulnerability.

ANXIETY DISORDERS Any disorder in which a person cannot control or resist the experience of anxiety. Examples include obsessions and compulsions, intrusive thoughts, hysterical reactions, all sorts of phobias, posttraumatic stress, and panic reactions.

ANXIETY DREAM See Dream theory, Freudian.

ANXIETY NEUROSIS Distress of anxiety pervades the personality and is consciously experienced. The anxiety is not limited to any specific target situation, nor is it converted into somatoform states—those resembling actual physical symptoms. Tension is experienced and therefore the anxiety is considered ego-dystonic or alien. Examples of such disorders include phobias and the traumatic disorders.

ANXIETY REACTION See Anxiety neurosis.

ANXIETY SENSITIVITY Tendency to exaggerate experience in the sense of expecting the worst to be the case. For example, a stomach ache can generate anxiety because the symptom of the stomach ache can be seen as either the harbinger of cancer, some prodromal indication of cancer, or as having actual cancer. Such anxiety sensitivity is generally correlated to a hypochondriacal condition.

APHASIA Disturbance in language and communication. This impairment results from a brain event. There are many variants of aphasia.

Expressive aphasia—an inability to utilize the necessary word or phrase in order to convey a thought. In the recovery process people begin to use synonyms when the word they are searching for eludes them.

Receptive aphasia—an inability to grasp another's communication.

APHONIA Muteness. Can be a conversion symptom.

APNEA See Sleep apnea.

APTITUDE TEST Designed to assess at what a person is best.

ARCHAIC EGO STATE The so-called oceanic feeling is frequently attributed to persons with this sort of psychic organization. Boundaries between the internal and external world seems absent in such a person's typical experience.

ARCHAIC THINKING Seen in psychosis, as in schizophrenia. Considered to be primitive thinking.

ARCHETYPE Jung's idea of a collective unconscious generates the concept of the archetype. It is a representation of specific prototypic styles—modes of thinking derived from the entire history of civilization.

ARIETI, SILVANO (1914–1981). European psychiatrist. Known for his work on schizophrenia, which is referred to as the trauma model of mental disorders.

ARLOW, JACOB (1912–2004). Influential American psychiatrist / psychoanalyst who, along with Charles Brenner, created interest in the arena of wishes as the focal point of psychoanalytic theory and was known for his contributions to the understanding of unconscious fantasy, empathy, the concept of time, and emotion.

AS-IF PERSONALITY Coined by Helene Deutsch (1884–1982), a European psychoanalyst, and used both by Adler and Sullivan to indicate a fantasized construction developed to elevate self-esteem. Considered by Freudians to be defined as a component of the compensatory defense. Such individuals behave *as if* they are in synchrony with the ideas and feelings they are propounding, but it is only the appearance of authenticity that exists. There is a thin diagnostic line between an as-if condition and one that is characterized by depersonalization or derealization. The as-if personality is considered to be a prepsychotic condition in which schizoid features such as an absence of warmth is noticed, although the as-if person can actually appear to be socially appropriate. This appearance of social normalcy is largely based upon mimicry. Chameleonlike behavior is typical for the as-if personality. Thus, it is the description of a person who has been taken over by artifice or persona needs, so that, in essence, the natural personality has been usurped. Such individuals have been characterized as inauthentic and to be constantly seeking consensus with others.

AS-IF TECHNIQUE Method used in George Kelly's fixed role therapy in which clients act in a way that is driven by assumptions about the world or themselves that are incongruent with their usual self-defeating beliefs.

ASPERGER'S SYNDROME Named for Hans Asperger, European physician (1844–1954). Considered high-level autism. Such people have savant abilities and often demonstrate high achievement. Various symptoms such as difficulty with eye contact as well as social inappropriateness are apparent. Underdevelopment of peer relationships is characteristic and emotional reciprocity is compromised. Language development is usually undisturbed and there is no apparent delay seen in cognitive development. Considered to be a pervasive developmental disorder in the *Diagnostic and Statistical Manual* of the American Psychiatric Association. See Pervasive developmental disorders.

ASSAGIOLI, ROBERTO See Psychosynthesis.

ASSERTIVENESS TRAINING Procedure used in cognitive behavior therapy designed to help clients practice expressing their wants and feelings in more adaptive ways. Usually involves cognitive restructuring, modeling, role-playing, feedback, relaxation, and other techniques.

ASSOCIATION A term used in psychoanalysis to mean connecting ideas in the absence of any real restriction. This is called free association. Also one of Bleuler's four *A*s, the impairment of which leads the clinician to consider possible contamination of the ego and schizophrenic thinking. See Free association.

ASSUMPTION GROUP Wilfred Bion's stunning theory regarding the three basic cultures (or underlying assumptions) of groups, which determine its chief emotions and motives and, in addition, characterize the essential resistance of the group.

The dependency group culture is one where the members look to the leader for security.

The pairing group culture is one in which the group looks to any two members who could comprise a couple and toward whom the entire group could amalgamate its hope.

The fight-flight group culture in which, if the members experience a lack of interest on the part of the therapist, it is then considered emotional abandonment and either the members continually attack the therapist or members studiously avoid interaction with one another.

ASTHENIC TYPE Term coined by Kretschmer depicting a thin and weak type of person. Similar to Sheldon's ectomorph. See Kretschmer, Emil.

ATTACHMENT Important concept in object relations theory and studied further by Bowlby, who demonstrated that there is actually a domain to attachment that includes all sorts of verbal as well as nonverbal signals regarding bonding, separation, and general communication. See Bowlby, Edward John Mostyn.

ATTENTION DEFICIT / HYPERACTIVITY DISORDER (ADHD) Afflicting children as well as adults. Difficulty in attention span, organization, and focus. Later in life results in trouble holding a job. In childhood, makes studying in school difficult. Important items needed to finish a job are often lost and, in addition, sustained activity is a challenge. Forgetfulness and distractibility are characteristic. Hyperactivity, restlessness, impulsivity, and impaired judgment are behaviors seen both in children and adults who suffer from this condition, as is fidgeting, excessive running and climbing, and impatience. Subject to treatment through medication such as amphetamines.

ATTRIBUTIONAL AMBIGUITY Referring to possible racial microaggression. Studied by Bucceri, Capodilupo, Esquilin, Holder, Nada, Sue, and Torino.

ATTRIBUTIONAL STYLE In cognitive behavioral therapy considered a typical tendency to attribute causes to events. Includes dimensions of

internal-external—events attributed to the self or to external stimuli;

stable-unstable—events attributed to more permanent causes or to temporary ones;

global-specific—events attributed to causes that generalize to several events or solely to one event.

AUDIBLE THOUGHT See Thought disorder.

AURA An odd feeling that precedes either an epileptic seizure or sick headaches.

AUTISM Considered a brain anomaly with a general withdrawal syndrome including idiosyncratic thinking. The person relies almost entirely on the internal signal for the pursuit of needs without particular attention to the external signals of objectivity or reality. Thought processes can be fractured and behavior can be unusual and anormal. In autistic children classic symptomatology includes difficulty in eye contact, arrested social development, and an inability to care for oneself—especially with respect to health habits. Speech prosody is disturbed. Pitch, volume, tonality, cadence are affected negatively and emerge as inappropriate. Peer relationships are underdeveloped and corresponding emotional reciprocity is absent. Spoken language is similarly underdeveloped and repetitive motor mannerisms are seen. Listed as a pervasive developmental disorder in the *Diagnostic and Statistical Manual* of the American Psychiatric Association.

AUTISTIC PHASE See Mahler, Margaret.

AUTOEROTICISM Usually meant to imply solipsistic sexuality. This means that the sexual impulse is informed within the context of the self, as in masturbation. A form of narcissistic preoccupation.

AUTOHYPNOSIS Self-induced trance.

AUTOMATIC BEHAVIOR Behavior in the absence of voluntary control.

AUTOMATIC THOUGHTS Habitual thoughts, often outside of immediate awareness, triggered by events or circumstances that influence emotions and behavior. In Beck's cognitive therapy a major aim is to recognize distorted thoughts and assumptions and replace them with other thoughts that are better validated and not self-defeating. See Cognitive specificity hypothesis.

AUTOMATIC WRITING The process of writing in the absence of consciousness of the activity or while the writer is in a trance. Writing under hypnosis. Reputed to reveal unconscious material.

AUTONOMIC NERVOUS SYSTEM (ANS) Aspect of the nervous system that controls bodily functions in the absence of consciousness. The usual example is one's heartbeat. The ANS consists of the sympathetic and parasympathetic nervous systems that together comprise the autonomic nervous system that regulates visceral and homeostatic systems of the body (heart, colon, bladder).

AUTONOMOUS EGO FUNCTION Considered by Hartmann to reflect high-level functioning in the absence of impulsive behavior. Impairment of the primary autonomous function of the ego reflects gross perceptual disturbance as well as a variety of other psychotic characteristics. Impairment of the secondary autonomous function of the ego indicates incipient schizophrenic process or borderline personality functioning. See Hartmann, Heinz.

AUTONOMY A concept specifically designed to reflect a sense that independent behavior, responsibility for the self, and living life in a way that demonstrates a growing up out of a dependent relationship (as in child to parent) characterizes the personality. Self-governing.

AUTOPLASTY Changing difficulties in one's world by changing the self. See Alloplasty.

AVERSION THERAPY Negative conditioning.

AVERSIVE CONDITIONING Therapeutic technique to help reduce an undesired behavior (e.g., alcohol or substance abuse) by pairing it with a noxious stimulus.

AWARENESS TECHNIQUE In Gestalt therapy individuals become aware of aspects of their expressive behavior such as body language, voice prosody, and emotions.

AWFULIZING AND ANTI-AWFULIZING In Ellis's rational emotive behavior therapy, a tendency to exaggerate the negative consequences of real or anticipated events (awfulizing) and the therapeutic attempt to counteract one's exaggerated negative thinking (anti-awfulizing). See Catastrophizing; Elegant REBT; Inelegant REBT.

AXIS I AND AXIS II In *DSM* nomenclature:

Axis I—contains all clinical psychological disorders that are not of the personality disorder type, such as the anxiety disorders.

Axis II—contains all of the personality disorders including paranoid, schizoid, schizotypal, antisocial, borderline, histrionic, narcissistic, avoidant, dependent, and obsessive-compulsive, in addition to the reportage of mental retardation as well as notation of defenses.

B

BAD OBJECT In psychoanalytic and object relations theory, this is the dynamic object—usually internal—that has malice toward the self. Originally, the good object was the nonsexual one, while the bad object was sexual. More modern terminological usage refers to the good object as a reference to the good parent or good parent transferential figure. The bad object refers to the internalized bad parent or bad parent transferential figure. May refer to either an internal or external object, but usually is used for the internal object. See Good object; Splitting.

BALINT, MICHAEL (1896–1970). European psychoanalyst/biochemist known as a British object relations theorist. Of his major contributions are included

Psychoanalytic theory—an object relations revision of psychoanalytic theory, especially with respect to psychosexual development and its implications for derivative functioning.

Primary narcissism—a revision of the nature of primary narcissism. He speaks of "primary love."

Character structure—a new look at the infrastructure of character formation.

Basic fault—the discrepancy between what the infant needed and what the primary caretaker was able to provide. Subject seeks primary object love—equivalent to unconditional love desired from the therapist. Thus a person's entire development contains false premises and faulty processes based upon seeing oneself as defective or damaged as a result of disturbed mother-infant bonding. In treatment the basic fault promotes a "malignant regression" as opposed to a "benign regression," leading to enactment through externalization and the avoidance of the experiencing of the primal trauma.

BANDURA, ALBERT (1925–). Canadian born American psychologist. Pioneer in social learning theory, adolescent aggression, and the role of observational learning.

Published classic texts on social cognitive theory and self efficacy.

BASIC ASSUMPTION GROUP Bionian formulation regarding the basic motive of the group along with its corresponding basic emotion. See Assumption group; Bion, Wilfred.

BASIC FAULT See Balint, Michael.

BASIC ID A diagnostic acronym used for assessment in the seven basic interactive areas of multimodal therapy introduced by psychologist Arnold Lazarus—describing seven basic domains of functioning: behaviors, affective responses, sensations, imagery, cognitions, interpersonal relationships, and (the need for) drugs or other biological interventions.

BASIC RULE The basic rules of the psychoanalytic process: that is, to reduce acting out by verbalizing tensions and to attempt to overcome resistance in order to surface repressed material. Accomplished by the assumption that the patient will tell the analyst everything that comes to mind.

BATTERED CHILD SYNDROME Typically, aggression toward the child is by the parent or caregiver, who is either physically punishing the child with beatings or aggressing toward the child with sexual attacks. Such children show borderline personality development along with depressive qualities.

BAYLEY SCALES OF INFANT AND TODDLER DEVELOPMENT Developmental scales for use with infants and children one month to three and one half years.

mental scale—assesses memory, perception, and learning;
motor scale—assesses motor abilities;
behavior rating scale—assesses behavior categories such as attention, orientation, and emotional regulation;
social emotional scale and adaptive scale—surveys parent perceptions of their child's development.

BECK, AARON T. (1921–). Influential analytically trained American psychiatrist who, in the early 1960s, originated cognitive therapy as a treatment for depression and developed depression and suicide assessment scales. With research purporting to refute the idea of introjected anger as the cause of depression, Beck demonstrated that depressed individuals hold certain negative biases about themselves, the world, and the future. Subsequently applied his approach to the treatment of anxiety and a host of other disorders. See Cognitive specificity hypothesis; Cognitive therapy; Negative automatic thoughts.

BECK DEPRESSION INVENTORY (BDI) Widely used instrument to assess depression.

BEEBE, BEATRICE (1946–). American psychologist/psychoanalyst who has provided consistent research in the field of early infant development, mother-infant interaction, and the origins of the processes of relatedness. Has mapped, along with Lachmann, the dyadic interaction that organizes self as well as the interactive processes in mothers and infants, with analogies for patients and analysts. The metapsychological umbrella of this work is comprised of systems theory, self psychology theory, intersubjective theory, and phenomenological relational theory more generally.

BEHAVIOR, CATASTROPHIC Behavior that reflects the person's inability to do something—a feeling of being overwhelmed is typical.

BEHAVIOR DISORDERS These are behaviors of children and adolescents who engage in acting out activities such as stealing, lying, temper tantrums, fighting, and setting fires. If chronic, implies a psychopathic diagnosis. The work of Stella Chess, among many others, represents a major focus on the vicissitudes of behavior disorders.

BEHAVIOR THERAPY Form of psychotherapy developed by Hans Eysenck (at the University of London), Joseph Wolpe, and others. Applies learning principles of operant conditioning and Pavlovian conditioning rather than the use of exploration of underlying psychological causes. Techniques include systematic desensitization, relaxation training, behavior rehearsal, modeling, flooding, and biofeedback.

BEHAVIORAL MEDICINE Behavioral and biomedical technology brought to bear on the treatment.

BEHAVIORAL REHEARSAL In cognitive and behavioral therapies, practicing interpersonal behavior until clients are able to implement them in real-life situations. See Assertiveness training; Role-play.

BEHAVIORISM J. B. Watson formulated this approach to psychology, which focuses on observable, quantitative events, positing that mental events, being subjective, are not scientifically verifiable. See Watson, John Broadus.

BELL OBJECT RELATIONS INVENTORY (BORI) Measures deficits in object relations ego functioning from an ego-psychological perspective. Includes a four factor scale of narcissism, shame, masochism, and object relations. Assesses interpersonal relatedness, diagnosis, and psychopathology.

BENDER, LAURETTA (1897–1987). American child neuropsychiatrist. Creator of the Bender Gestalt Visual Motor Test. This paper and pencil test requires the subject to replicate geometric figures and is utilized in the diagnosis of brain disorders and personality tendencies.

BENDER GESTALT VISUAL MOTOR TEST Part of the standard clinical test battery.

BERNE, ERIC (1910–1970). Canadian psychiatrist. See Transactional analysis.

BETTELHEIM, BRUNO (1903–1990). European American child psychologist. A controversial figure insofar as his insistence that autism is a function primarily of a "refrigerator mother" supported by an "absentee father" has been decisively discredited by modern studies of brain disease and brain anomalies. Well known for his books "*Uses of Enchantment* and *The Empty Fortress.*

BIOBEHAVIORAL SHIFT At about three months of age the infant shows a quantum leap in development, as in, for example, an improved ability to tolerate frustration.

BIOENERGETICS A body-focused therapy developed by Lowen and influenced by Reich. See Body-focused therapy.

BIOFEEDBACK Use of an external monitoring device (GSR, EMG, or pulse rate) to enhance relaxation training and control of autonomic functions and, after therapeutic interventions, to monitor changes in clients' responses to aversive mental or physical stimuli.

BION, WILFRED (1897–1979). Psychoanalyst born in India and educated in England. See Assumption Group.

BIPOLAR DISORDER Referring to the affect disorders of mania and depression as separate episodic experiences in the unipolar sense, and also as part of a manic-depressive sequence.

Type I—refers to severe manic episodes.

Type II—includes episodes of depression along with a history of hypomania (a condition not quite manic, although excited). *Cyclothymic disorder*—is also included within the Type II category although here, the manic-like state exists in the form of elation, while the depression-like state exists in the form of dejection.

Bipolar disorder can also contain a psychotic cast with features such as a display by the subject of exceedingly stubborn resistance to instructions or requests. Excessive motor activity along with intermittent severe inertia can also be typical. A catatoniclike excitement resulting from sudden upsurges of frustration and anger are also possible, so that the subject can become dangerously impulsive and even violent. Such outbursts will always prevail over considered judgment.

BIRTH TRAUMA Concept promoted by Otto Rank suggesting that the trauma of birth is the precursor to anxiety and psychopathology.

BIZARRENESS A term used clinically to indicate inappropriate, odd, and what would be considered weird behavior. Usually cited in cases of schizophrenic behavior that is wildly out of keeping with reality signals.

BLEULER, EUGEN (1857–1939). European psychiatrist who pioneered definitions and clinical criteria for the assessment of schizophrenia. See Schizophrenia.

BLINDNESS, HYSTERICAL A form of hysterical symptomatology defined as conversion hysteria.

BODY DYSMORPHIC DISORDER Imagined (delusional) defect in appearance.

BODY EGO See Ego, body.

BODY-FOCUSED THERAPY Conceptualization of psychological therapy as necessitating physical release of tension and emotion through physical manipulation, massage, and even martial arts. Such therapy includes yoga, Feldenkrais method, Rolfing, bioenergetics, and Alexander Technique.

BOLLAS, CHRISTOPHER (1944–). British school of object relations. Bollas has created a new glossary of concepts that he applies to the experience of subjects in their world. These include memories of infancy and childhood—of primary object figures, the self among them. Some terms of this glossary include

cast a shadow—the object can "cast a shadow," which essentially affects the child;
cracking up—breaking up streams of consciousness;
idiom—subject's idiosyncratic context: the core of the self (even operating at birth);
normotic illness—transforming language to render it incomprehensible;
sudden catastrophic disillusion—absolute disbelief;
suspended attentiveness—the analyst's stance;
transformational object relationship—child's entitled feeling for having access to the primary object;
unthought known—a traumatic experience is split off from consciousness so that it is known but not thought;
violent innocents—people who disavow their own perception of reality (especially if it is troubling), with violent consequences.

See Object relations theory.

BORDERLINE INTELLIGENCE Historically considered to be an IQ (intelligence quotient) about twenty points below the average score of 100.

BORDERLINE PERSONALITY Unfortunate term in clinical usage because it implies a border condition between normalcy and psychosis or between neurosis and psychosis—a fact accepted by various clinicians. Yet the borderline condition has been identified more as a personality disorder that includes features such as poor inner controls, a thin ego (meaning poor resilience of the ego), a hair-trigger tendency to experience anger and to act it out, suicidal gestures, addictive activity, poor sense of self, a tendency to both idealize and devalue significant others, episodes of impaired reality testing temporarily based upon the person's strong sense of wishes (along with a corresponding inability to integrate disappointment of such wishes), a marked foreboding of vulnerability, and a prevailing sense of aloneness. Psychotherapy is very difficult, largely because of the plethora of symptoms and the issue of both idealizing and devaluing the therapist in the face of such poor frustration tolerance. Yet fears of abandonment prevail, and other problematic symptoms can include self-mutilation behavior, suicidal ideation and gestures, recklessness, and paranoid and dissociative behavior. The so-called high functioning borderline personality is one who, although suffering with the entire borderline syndrome, nevertheless demonstrates a firmer ego (less thin) and is therefore able to function more normally. In the psychiatric nomenclature the borderline is considered a personality disorder, not a psychosis. Theoreticians of the borderline personality include Gabbard, Giovacchini, Gunderson, Kernberg, Linehan, Masterson, and A. Wolberg.

BOUNDARY, EGO A clinical concept used in its general sense to distinguish between the inner life and external reality. In a more specific clinical sense the inner ego boundary is designed to keep repressed material contained in repression, while the outer ego boundary is designed in the psyche to keep the ego free from contaminated external signals.

BOWLBY, EDWARD JOHN MOSTYN (1907–1990). British psychiatrist/psychoanalyst who developed what is known as attachment theory. He integrated evolutionary biology, psychoanalysis, and cognitive science to bring the issue of childcaregiver attachment phenomena to bear on mental health and, at the same time, minimized Freudian instinct theory as crucial to the development of the infant. Instead, Bowlby focused on the importance of the infant-caretaker bond and its appropriateness to the needs of the infant. This is considered a focus on object relations within the context of a self-psychological perspective. His work supports Melanie Klein's view that mourning is a natural and necessary phenomenon in human development.

BRAIN DISORDER Usually refers to organic brain syndrome. In a clinical test such as the Bender Gestalt Visual Motor Test, as well as with respect to clinical behavior, a person diagnosed with the general state of organic brain syndrome will show signs of poor frustration tolerance, impulsive behavior, quickness to anger, and concreteness. In replicating the geometric figures of the test, subjects will draw the figures in a way that demonstrates "collisions" between the shapes—clinically reflecting the state of the subjects' organizational incapacity, impulsivity, and poor overall control.

BRAIN, EMOTIONAL In the domain of neuropsychoanalysis, the R prefrontal cortex is seen as essential to motivation, intuition, emotionally centered cognitions, self-awareness, and empathy. This is the internal organizing agency and, according to Solms, is the thinking part of the emotional brain. According to Schore, the right brain emotional processes are essential to development, psychopathology, and psychotherapy. The right hemispheric dominance for affective states is largely responsible for attachment functions, object relational transactions, and affect-regulating defenses, such as dissociation.

BRENNER, CHARLES (1914–2008). American psychiatrist/psychoanalyst. Known for his classic text in psychoanalytic theory, *An Elementary Textbook of Psychoanalysis*, as well as his writing with respect to psychoanalytic technique. Along with Jacob Arlow, responsible for developing the alternative to id/superego conflict—namely, a focus on the conflict inherent in the vicissitudes of wishes. Also known for his work in affect theory and compromise formations. A pillar of the New York Psychoanalytic Institute. Founded in 1911 by Abraham A. Brill, the New York Psychoanalytic Institute housed a who's who faculty in psychoanalytic education. A sampling of luminaries through the almost century-long history of the institute include Arlow, Brenner, Peter Gay, Heinz Hartmann, Edith Jacobson,

Ernst Kris, Kurt Eissler, Margaret Mahler, Sandor Lorand, Sandor Rado, and Paul Schilder.

BREUER, JOSEPH (1842–1925). European physician / neurologist with whom Freud worked on cases of hysteria.

BRIDGING In the tradition of cognitive behavioral therapy, a way of moving from a deeply ingrained old belief to a new, more adaptive belief by making a key statement that produces a dramatic conceptual shift. Also a multimodal therapy technique in which therapy focuses first on the client's preferred modality (e.g., emotions) and later on other aspects the therapist may consider more basic, such as cognitions or behavior.

BRIEF PSYCHOTIC DISORDER See Brief reactive psychosis.

BRIEF REACTIVE PSYCHOSIS A breakdown of reality testing occurs in response to overwhelming external trauma. Recovery is expected within some weeks of the trauma. Equivalent to Brief psychotic disorder.

BULIMIA NERVOSA Eating disorder. Binge eating usually followed by depressive mood. Seen in young women beginning during adolescence, possibly continuing into adulthood. Binge eating is frequently followed by purging (vomiting), and this is noted in the *Diagnostic and Statistical Manual of Mental Disorders* as the purging type. To reduce weight, the nonpurging type will engage in excessive exercise and fasting.

BURRY, ANTHONY (1939–). American psychologist / psychoanalyst. Author of volumes in psychodiagnosis, differential diagnosis, and psychopathology. Member, editorial board, *Dictionary of Psychopathology.*

C

CAMISOLE Technical term for straight-jacket restraint. Camisoles were frequently used in mental hospitals up to the mid twentieth century to restrain out-of-control or rageful patients. As newer medications became available, the use of camisoles ceased.

CANCRO, ROBERT (1932–). American psychiatrist widely known for work in schizophrenia, psychopharmacology, psychopathology, diagnosis, and in the treatment of a wide variety of disorders (i.e., attention deficit, posttraumatic stress). Member, editorial board, *Dictionary of Psychopathology.*

CASTRATION ANXIETY A concept popularized by Freud to indicate a boy's apprehension about injury to or actual castration of the penis. In Freud's psychosexual stages the castration anxiety drama is seen in the oedipal phase in which the threat of castration ostensibly motivates resolution of the oedipal problem. As an acculturated derivative, and according to Kellerman, a gender difference seems to appear insofar as men defend against inferiority feelings by not tolerating humiliation (castration derivative). On the other hand, in order for women to defend against feelings of inferiority, being wrong (castration derivative) is difficult to tolerate. In contrast, women manage humiliation better, while men are generally less concerned about being wrong. In men, being humiliated is to finally be wrong or inferior, while in women, being wrong is to be humiliated and therefore inferior. Psychoanalytically then, derivatives of castration anxiety appear manifestly different by gender although from a psychoanalytic point of view, identical in underlying meaning.

CATALEPSY Refers to a patient remaining in any given postural position in the context of a condition known as waxy flexibility. Thus, the posture can be changed and the new position will then remain fixed indefinitely, only to be capable of changing again. Seen in patients diagnosed as schizophrenic–catatonic. See Schizophrenia.

CATAPLEXY A condition of a loss of voluntary musculature so that the sufferer then falls to the ground losing physical control of the self. In such a state, however, the person retains full consciousness. This cataplectic attack is usually seen as one of the tetrad of symptoms in narcoleptic states. The accompanying symptoms of the narcoleptic include the narcoleptic sleep state itself, hypnagogic hallucinations, and sleep paralysis. See Narcolepsy.

CATASTROPHIC BEHAVIOR See Behavior, catastrophic.

CATASTROPHIZING A concept utilized in rational emotive behavior therapy to reveal the distortion made by people who are presented with a challenge and imagine the worst that can possibly happen to them with respect to such a situation. See Awfulizing and Anti-awfulizing.

CATATONIA A form of schizophrenia in which the patient variably demonstrates periods of stupor, as well as periods of excitement. Includes cataleptic attacks. See Schizophrenia.

CATHARSIS A concept developed by Freud. In modern usage it is seen as the state in which a patient, through the talking method, and by getting things off his chest, will feel better. Known psychoanalytically, as getting better through abreaction.

CATHEXIS Psychic investment of energy in some object—either a self representation, or an object in the world such as a person, or even an idea, or symbol. A salient psychoanalytic precept.

CBT See Cognitive behavior therapy.

CHARACTER Frequently used interchangeably with *personality.* Yet, personality is the more inclusive term, implying, under its psychological umbrella, levels and aspects of the person. These include diagnostic syndromes, psychophysiological reactions, functional symptoms, the organization of defense mechanisms, emotions and their relation to traits, cognitive style, psychodynamics, and so forth. In contrast, *character* most often refers to character structure. Character is not meant to imply the nature of any particular moral fiber or ethics. Character has a clinical meaning and refers to the organization of character traits and typical behaviors of the personality. According to the early psychoanalytic pioneer, Wilhelm Reich, character refers to anxiety in the personality that is bound—the organization of personality traits are tightly woven in order to tame or neutralize anxiety. Thus, individuals with character disorders are those who show no anxiety or where the tension is ego-syntonic (not experienced), in contrast to the neuroses, or anxiety disorders, where tension or anxiety is ego-alien or dystonic (experienced). See Character defense.

CHARACTER DEFENSE Those defense mechanisms that are directed toward the elimination of anxiety so that the personality profile is free of the conscious experience of anxiety. Examples are

internalization—of rules and regulations;
introjection—of attitudes and identifications;
splitting—that is, parsing the good from the bad.

CHARACTER DISORDER See Personality / character disorder.

CHARACTER RESISTANCE The system of defense that is developed to support the character structure—the way a person is.

CHARACTER STRUCTURE Etched behavioral patterns of the personality that developed to avoid anxiety. Composed of set personality patterns.

CHARCOT, JEAN-MARTIN (1825–1893). French psychiatrist and neurologist well known in psychoanalytic lore for his work with hypnosis and conversion hysteria and, of course, in his association with Freud.

CHIA Children's Inventory of Anger based on rational emotive behavior therapy.

CHILD AND ADOLESCENT PSYCHOTHERAPY See Developmental psychology.

CHILDHOOD DISINTEGRATIVE DISORDER A diagnosis within the category designated as a pervasive developmental disorder. In this category the child begins to lose capacity before age ten. This loss of capacity can be in expressive or receptive language, social skills, general adaptive behavior, stereotyped mannerisms, bladder control, aspects of play, and motor skills.

CHODOROW, NANCY (1944–). American humanist, leading theorist in feminist thought, psychoanalytic sociologist, and proponent of object relations theory. Respects work of Horney, M. Klein, Loewald, and Slater.

CHROMATIC: ACHROMATIC Affect ratio. See Rorschach Test.

CIRCADIAN RHYTHM Refers to the natural biological cycle of about twenty-four hours.

CIRCADIAN RHYTHM SLEEP DISORDER Equivalent to sleep-wake schedule disorder. See Sleep disorders; Dyssomnia; Parasomnia.

CIRCUMPLEX ORGANIZATION A graphic representation of any universe of clinical relationships, e.g., emotions, traits, diagnoses. These are arranged in quadrants divided by two independent perpendicular axes of polar opposite terms, e.g., active-passive and dependent-independent. All terms within the circle are thereby correlated so that those closest are most similar, while those furthest apart are less similar. The resulting organization of terms comprise a similarity structure.

CIRCUMSTANTIAL THINKING A disturbance of association in schizophrenia where the person will not get to the point: the central idea is lost in a sea of tangents and in irrelevant detail.

CLANG ASSOCIATION Selection of words based on similarity of sound and not on meaning. Seen in disturbances of association in schizophrenia as well as in affective psychoses.

CLAUSTROPHOBIA Involuntary fear of closed spaces. Freud said, "Behind the fear is the wish." See Phobia; Symptom.

CLIENT-CENTERED THERAPY See Rogers, Carl

CLINICAL PSYCHOLOGY A broad field in which, with respect to psychotherapy and the study of psychopathology, the psychologist is generally trained in psychodynamic psychology or in cognitive behavioral psychology as well as in a host of other treatment modalities. Psychodiagnostic testing as well as personality interpretation through a variety of projective and objective tests is also a specialty. The clinical psychologist can also apply expertise in any number of psychological consultations, from forensic work to work with a wide variety of clinical populations. The clinical psychologist is also trained in experimental lab techniques. Clinical psychologists hold either the Ph.D. or Psy.D. degrees.

CLOSURE In clinical usage the seeking of finality to any project. Individuals who are frequently anxious or even compulsive are usually occupied with activity that consistently becomes fueled by motivation toward this sort of "closing" endeavor. During this period of awaiting closure, such individuals are permeated with fantasy that includes tension regarding the delay in finding closure as well as the tension that exists during the pursuit of closure itself.

CLUSTER HEADACHE See Headache, cluster.

CLUTTERING Frequently unintelligible speech as a result of rapid-fire talking along with incorrect phrasing and staccato cadence. In the psychiatric nomenclature it is considered to be a specific developmental disorder and, as such, is considered to be a language and speech disorder.

CODEPENDENCY Excessive caring for another, psychodynamically attributed to the need for control as well as signifying appeasement behavior.

COGNITION Distinct from emotion and referring to higher mental processes such as perceiving, knowing, evaluating, reasoning, remembering, and problem solving. Largely consciously based.

COGNITIVE-AFFECTIVE CROSSFIRE The contrast between cognitive and affective responses to others' feedback as these affect people's views of themselves.

COGNITIVE ANXIETY Event-related experience of worry and tension.

COGNITIVE APPRAISAL THERAPY Proposed by Richard Lazarus; posits that cognitive assessment is implicitly involved in all emotional reactions. Considered an aspect of cognitive motivational relational theory.

COGNITIVE AROUSAL THEORY OF EMOTION Developed by Schachter and Singer; proposes that emotional states derive from physiological arousal along with cognitive interpretations of the physical state. See Schachter, Stanley.

COGNITIVE BEHAVIOR MODIFICATION Approach developed by psychologist Donald Meichenbaum; cognitive stress inoculation training, which emphasizes conceptualization and structure as playing an important role in helping clients understand the change process prior to treatment.

COGNITIVE BEHAVIOR THERAPY (CBT) Beck's cognitive therapy, Ellis's rational-emotive behavior, and related approaches whose primary emphasis is on identifying and challenging illogical and self-defeating beliefs, rather than underlying psychodynamic constructs, as a means of changing maladaptive feelings and behavior. CBT approaches emphasize the interrelationships of thoughts, feelings, and behavior and utilize a wide range of techniques including disputation and restructuring of irrational beliefs, imagery, problem solving, behavioral rehearsal, emotive-expressive techniques, and relaxation practice. Therapists and clients collaborate in setting and monitoring goals, and therapy generally occurs over a relatively short-term period.

COGNITIVE CLICK Clients' "aha" experience or a cognitive synthesis during which it crystallizes that problems have ensued from faulty thinking and that this thinking must be altered in order to effect change.

COGNITIVE CLOSURE Seeing and understanding the entire picture of something.

COGNITIVE CONDITIONING A kind of negative conditioning designed to cure untoward behavior, e.g., a client repeatedly imagines vomit in a glass of alcohol until the thought discourages the behavior. See Conditioned response.

COGNITIVE CONSONANCE Two cognitive elements are consistent with one another and one can follow the other in a logically consecutive manner. See Cognitive dissonance theory.

COGNITIVE CONTINUUM In cognitive behavior therapy, this is a continuum that enables one to trace the shift from absolutistic core beliefs to those that are less absolute, thereby revealing that the individual is actually progressing with respect to altering a variety of distortions held within the core belief system. See Core belief.

COGNITIVE DECONSTRUCTION Concrete focus on sensation and immediate stimuli along with a conspicuous absence of affect. Thought to be a strategy of escape from conflict and trauma.

COGNITIVE DERAILMENT Schizophrenic thinking in which shifting of thoughts create illogical sequences.

COGNITIVE DISSONANCE THEORY Two cognitive elements are inconsistent with one another, resulting in an unpleasant psychological state. Attempts to reduce the discomfort include suppressing awareness of elements creating the conflict. First described by Leon Festinger. See Festinger, Leon.

COGNITIVE DISTORTIONS Systematic errors in perceiving and evaluating people and situations. Typical distortions identified by cognitive therapy pioneer Aaron T. Beck include all-or-nothing thinking, overgeneralization, emotional reasoning, and mental filter. In Ellis's REBT, distorted or irrational thinking is characterized by "shoulding," "awfulizing," global self or other rating, and "I-can't-stand-it-it is." See Automatic thoughts; Cognitive restructuring; Irrational beliefs.

COGNITIVE FLOODING Cognitive behavioral therapy treatment of phobia or trauma that focuses the client's imaginal experiencing of anxiety-generating situations, then introducing relaxation, imagery, or other methods to reduce the feelings of anxiety.

COGNITIVE GENERALIZATION Analogous to transfer of training; the ability to utilize knowledge in one area and apply it to problems in other areas.

COGNITIVE LOAD Extent of mental challenges or demands. See Cognitive overload.

COGNITIVE MAPS Core schemas acquired through experience and observation. These are mediated through symbolism and meaning that serve as the lens through which people view themselves and the world.

COGNITIVE MEDIATION Intervening variable between stimulus and response.

COGNITIVE MISER Person who seeks expedient solutions rather than more thoughtful ones. Parsimony rather than patience fills the need, and impulse triumphs over delay. In psychodynamic understanding, analogous to the issue of frustration tolerance, expecially with respect to urgent compensatory needs.

COGNITIVE NARROWING Focusing only on part of a situation or task rather than the whole.

COGNITIVE OVERLOAD Demands of a situation exceed a person's mental abilities to cope with it. See Cognitive load.

COGNITIVE PENETRABILITY Mental processes become influenced by the person's existing beliefs, knowledge, or goals (as opposed to reflexes).

COGNITIVE REHEARSAL Client imagines anxiety-laden situations, then develops and rehearses positive coping statements that will ultimately result in more adaptive feelings and behavior.

COGNITIVE RESTRUCTURING Cognitive behavior therapy technique for correcting distorted and maladaptive perceptions, beliefs, and cognitions in order to effect changes in emotions and behaviors.

COGNITIVE SCHEMA See Schema.

COGNITIVE SLIPPAGE Loosening of associations seen in schizophrenic individuals.

COGNITIVE SPECIFICITY HYPOTHESIS Diagnoses or feeling states such as depression and anxiety that are associated with certain kinds of automatic thoughts. See Negative automatic thoughts.

COGNITIVE STYLE The characteristic manner in which a person perceives, thinks, and solves problem. Styles can vary along a continuum, as, for example, preferences for visual as against verbal coding, individual as against group activity, structured as against open-ended situations, reflectivity as against impulsivity.

COGNITIVE TASK ANALYSIS Identifying the cognitive processes involved in the performance of a task.

COGNITIVE THERAPY Approach originated by American psychiatrist Aaron T. Beck, based on the theory that dysfunctional emotions and behaviors result from distorted beliefs and cognitions about oneself and others. Through guiding clients first to identify their distorted perceptions and cognitions and then change them to more logical ones (cognitive restructuring), therapists can significantly help reduce emotional disturbance and generate more adaptive behavior. See Cognitive Behavior Therapy (CBT).

COGNITIVE TRIAD See Negative triad.

COGNITIVE UNCONSCIOUS In cognitive psychology or cognitive behavior therapy, mental processes that are inferred because of the presence of automaticity, habit, or grammatical rules. Contrasted to psychoanalytic notion of the unconscious, which involves material that is repressed to avoid anxiety, shame, guilt, or anger. See Tacit knowledge.

COGNITIVE VULNERABILITY Beliefs that, according to cognitive behavior therapy, increase the probability of depression. It is the belief that one needs a stronger person on whom to rely in order to survive and be happy and that seeking perfection brings security and self-worth.

COITUS Penile-vaginal intercourse.

COLD COGNITION In cognitive behavior therapies, refers to a mental processing of tasks or circumstances that does not involve feelings or emotions. See Hot cognition.

COLLECTIVE UNCONSCIOUS Jung's conception of historical/genetic imperatives that are etched in the so-called culture of the personality. The amalgamated sociocultural values handed down generationally and affecting the behavior and attitudes of people who exist within that particular society. Jung's "personal unconscious" refers to repressed psychical material, while the "collective unconscious" refers to psychical products that are presumably genetically based and inherited.

COMPANION, IMAGINARY Seen in children who create an imaginary friend. This friend or companion is trusted and trustworthy, and the child will share with this friend all sorts of secrets. Derived from a need for intimacy and sharing and considered to be a normal phenomenon of the fantasy life.

COMPARTMENTALIZATION A defense strategy of the psyche that parses aspects of psychological life for the purpose of keeping threatening material away from consciousness and protecting, thereby, against the experience of anxiety. Such threatening feelings frequently refer to angry feelings being kept unconscious, out of awareness, attributed to another, or kept in a separate and sealed compartment: in this way behavior can occur without interference from the consciousness of one's own guilt, shame, or anger toward a target person. Thus compartmentalization can even permit impulsive behavior to occur through the control of aspects of the personality. Related to the defense of isolation of affect, to obsessive mechanisms of defense, and crucial in the dynamic of the dissociated identity disordered personality.

COMPENSATION Usually referring to defense mechanisms. Designed to compensate—in the sense of elevating—

for feelings of despair, inadequacy, or inferiority complexes. The compensatory defense is also utilized in an attempt to manage depression. Considered an ego defense. In addition, compensatory behavior is seen in individuals who are narcissistically given to grandiosity and will become oppositional whenever they find themselves in social situations where they feel subverted by others or, for whatever reason, not in a leadership position. They can thus feel undervalued and compelled to attack the real leader, even if the attack requires the dissemination of false information. In this sense, the attack on the leader becomes a form of character assassination, and this compensatory, oppositional, narcissistic, and grandiose attack is designed to gain social ascendancy and is done with characteristic and apparent dramatic sincerity.

COMPLEX Usually considered to be an amalgam of related ideas and feelings that are automatic (meaning repressed) but that influence the individual to behave in particular ways.

COMPLEX, CASTRATION A popularized Freudian notion that posits fear of losing the penis. See Castration anxiety.

COMPLEX, ELECTRA Essentially the Oedipus complex on the female side, reflecting the alliance (sexual or otherwise) between daughter and father. See Complex, Oedipus.

COMPLEX, INFERIORITY Referring to one's sense of worthlessness, weakness, and failure as compared to others. Compensatory mechanisms are usually seen in the behavior of individuals who experience inferiority feelings.

COMPLEX, MEDEA Hatred of mother toward child.

COMPLEX, OEDIPUS See Oedipus complex.

COMPLIMENTARITY Generally a family therapy concept, but also usually referring to the balance of forces between couples, or among groups of people, so that a reasonable homeostasis of the relationship obtains.

COMPROMISE FORMATION The appearance of a particular behavior or psychological phenomenon as a substitute for a primary or source underlying conflict. Therefore, a psychological / emotional symptom might be a good example of such a compromise formation—presumably expressing some portion of both sides of a conflict—superego restrictions versus the press of drives. In this sense, the compromise formation is also understood to affect the formation of character structure as in the reinforcement and fortification of trait behavior. See Symptom.

COMPULSION A behavior that the person feels must be done. Usually arises from an obsession (idea) about what must be done and culminates in the behavior of urgency in getting it done (action)—the compulsion itself. See Obsession.

COMPULSIVE MASTURBATION See Masturbation.

COMPULSIVE PERSONALITY Such a person seeks structure and standards by which to calibrate behavior and is generally underexpressive, strict in moral judgments, and given to rote work. Because of the need to be kept to standards, such a person may be quite sacrificial toward others by doing work for them—at times not even requested by the other. Gratification occurs in seeking and attaining closure. The compulsive person feels a compelling need to carry out an action that is frequently the end result of an obsession. From a psychoanalytic point of view, the compulsive act prevents forbidden thoughts to enter consciousness and thus the compulsive behavior, in characteristic fashion, supports repression. Such individuals are understood to be repressing anger. As a result, the compulsive behavior remains relatively free of anxiety and is thus ego-syntonic. See Ego-syntonic.

COMPULSIVE TALKING The need to hold forth in any verbal or social interaction. A key characteristic of such behavior concerns the person's inclination to keep talking while making no distinction between more or less important subject matter. There are essentially two types of compulsive talking:

Compulsive talking of the anxiety neurotic type—here the person will exhibit an inexorable need to control any conversation by regaling the listener(s) with a stream of consciousness usually in a dramatic (somewhat hysterical) manner punctuated by quick staccato laughter. The laughter is designed to invite the other(s) in on the assumption that what is being said is important and interesting. Frequently, the material is neither important nor interesting, but the laughter tends to mesmerize the listener(s) into believing that the subject matter discussed is, in fact, interesting. This kind of need to be at the center of things belies an anxious and depressive underlay. This particular compulsive talking symptom is nonpsychotic.

Compulsive talking of manic depressive psychosis—here the incessant talking is characterized by flat affect. Thus, where there are distinctions to be made between important and less important subject matter, the compulsive talker's affect contributes nothing to the listener's ability to distinguish what, in fact, is more or less important. In addition, such a person does not engage in this sort of incessant talking because of needs to be seen and central. Rather, the symptom is a function of a characterological manic syndrome presumably and simply designed to ward off the manifestations of underlying depression.

See Mania.

CONCRETE THINKING Referring to literal thinking in contrast to abstract thought. Severe concretization is seen in schizophrenic individuals who demonstrate paralogical or syncretistic thinking; that is, substituting correlational events for cause and effect.

CONCRETISTIC THINKING See Syncretistic thinking.

CONCRETIZATION A focus on detail and denotative meaning rather than on the abstract.

CONDENSATION Many ideas can be fused or condensed into a tighter package. One of Freud's dreamwork mechanisms, along with secondary elaboration, displacement, and symbolization.

CONDITIONED RESPONSE In Pavlovian conditioning, the learned response to a stimulus.

CONDITIONED STIMULUS A secondary stimulus that is paired with the primary stimulus so that contact with the secondary stimulus evokes the same response as the one to the original stimulus.

CONDITIONING Pavlovian term referring to the probability of a response becoming more or less likely depending on whether it is positively or negatively reinforced.

CONDITIONING, AVERSIVE See Aversive conditioning.

CONDITIONING, COGNITIVE See Cognitive conditioning.

CONDUCT DISORDERS These are behavior disorders of childhood involving aggressive and/or delinquent behavior.

CONFABULATION In order to fill in the gaps in one's memory or logic, phantasmagorical material can be inserted into percepts. Seen in patients with organic brain trauma and used conceptually in Rorschach (ink blot) assessment to indicate faulty thinking as expressed in pathological verbalization and, in particular combinations of responses on the test itself. Also understood in neuropsychoanalysis as the subject sustaining distorted or false reality testing. Considered to be a reflection of a brain lesion in a region where emotion influences decision making.

CONFIGURATION A concept in gestalt psychology to indicate the cohesive extent of a group.

CONFLICT In psychoanalysis conflict can be identified and understood with reference to Freud's six basic theories as presented by Greenspan.

1. *adaptive theory*—concerns stressors on the ego with respect to reality testing and attempts to support secondary process in the face of frustration, anger, loss, and depression;
2. *economic theory*—concerns drives that aim to gain expression in consciousness and then ultimately in behavior and the forces of the personality that attempt to control such drives;
3. *genetic theory*—posits that conflict can result in the resistance that patients have to connecting current behavior with historical events;
4. *intrapsychic theory*—that of id and superego and the role of ego in the balance of these forces;
5. *psychosexual theory*—concerns issues that become fixated or fixed at various stages of development—oral, anal, phallic, oedipal;

6. *topographical theory*—of ideation and impulse, existing either in the unconscious, preconscious, or conscious part of the psyche, and the defensive structure designed to manage such material—especially when keeping such material in the unconscious is experienced intuitively as an imperative.

CONFLICT, BASIC Competition between different forces of the self. Developed by Horney.

CONFLICT, CENTRAL Difference between how the person really is (the real self) in contrast to the person's posturing. Developed by Horney.

CONFLICT-FREE AREA OF THE EGO In the midst of a typically busy ego, this is an area of the ego that is relatively tranquil or conflict free.

CONFLUENCE A term used by Adler to imply an epigenetic phenomenon in which biological givens of the personality await their environmental stimuli in order for a particular behavior or attitude to appear.

CONFUSIONAL STATE Depersonalization or derealization occurs as a result of an acute stressor.

CONIGLIARO, VINCENZO (1928–). Italian-born American psychiatrist / psychoanalyst. Specialist in psychotherapy education. Author of a volume on the use of dreams in psychodynamic psychotherapy. Founder, dean, and medical director, Training Institute for Mental Health. Member, editorial board, *Dictionary of Psychopathology.*

CONJOINT MARITAL THERAPY Both spouses seen together by the same therapist.

CONJUNCTIVE VARIABLE Essentially synonymous with the concept of an emulsifying agent—that variable which, when introduced into a situation, will create harmony. Developed by Sullivan.

CONNECTIONISM In cognitive psychology, the mind seen as a network of units.

CONSCIENCE In psychoanalysis, equivalent to the superego: that which produces guilt and stands in opposition to the dangers of impulse expression. Correlated to moral and ethical imperatives.

CONSCIOUSNESS Awareness: in psychoanalytic metapsychology correlated to secondary process. See Limbic system.

CONSTANCY Referring to stability of trait characteristics. In object relations theory constancy refers to inner or internalized objects that remain stable and reliable even in the face of everyday challenges.

CONTAMINATION Mixing parts of words so that a schizophrenic underlay seems diagnostically credible. In Rorschach (ink blots) such percepts are correspondingly seen to be pathognomonic (major variable) of psychosis.

CONTENT In dreams, Freud refers to two levels of content:

the manifest level—the descriptive dream itself;
the latent level—the underlying or more primary unraveled part of the dream that can be accessed by analysis of associations to certain elements of the manifest dream.

CONTEXTUALISM The totality of any experience is as important as any detail of the experience.

CONTEXTUALIST PERSPECTIVE In intersubjectivity theory, refers to the complex mixture of forces that shape any interpersonal interaction. See Stolorow, Robert.

CONTINUITY THEORY Usually refers to prediction of life's influence on aging. Continuity theory holds that past is prologue so that how you have behaved, more or less, will determine how you will behave. Alternatively, life-event-stress theory emphasizes that individual signal events have greater impact in determining how a person will behave in later life.

CONTROL Usually considered a measure of maturity, especially in contrast with the nature and amount of impulse. Assessed on the Rorschach Test. Of course an overabundance of control features of the personality can reveal an obsessive, compulsive, rather rigid and inflexible approach to intrapersonal dynamics and interpersonal events.

CONTROL ANALYSIS A psychoanalyst in training undergoing personal psychoanalysis. Along with this, the psychoanalyst who is treating a patient is supervised by another psychoanalyst in order to scrutinize the treatment for the purpose of training.

CONVERSION AND CONVERSION HYSTERIA Indicates a physical manifestation (symptom) caused by a psychological/emotional state (repressed emotion). Thus considered to be a symptom with symbolic meaning inherent in such a physical manifest symptom. In conversion hysteria the subject is frequently indifferent to the symptom—as in *la belle indifference.*

COPING Usually refers to coping mechanisms, as in the ability to adapt or accommodate to challenges the person experiences. Also commonly equates with defense and defense mechanisms.

CORE BELIEF In cognitive behavior therapy, core belief systems or schemas about the self, others, and the world that keep the individual locked into anxiety, depression, anger, guilt, or other dysfunctional emotions; relates to poor self and other acceptance; and relates also to avoidant or other self-defeating behavior. See Schema.

CORRECTIVE EMOTIONAL EXPERIENCE The working through of conflict in the psychoanalytic process by virtue of the interaction between patient and therapist so that, in the present, childhood conflicts are no longer persuasive with respect to how they previously had been as the determiners of automatic reactions.

CORRELATIONAL THINKING See Syncretistic thinking.

COTHERAPY Refers to two therapists together conducting group therapy.

COUNSELING Equivalent to mentoring and implying less than an in-depth therapeutic investigation. Useful for vocational, guidance, school problems, spiritual guidance, and marital intervention.

COUNTERCATHEXIS Investment in defense systems to support resistance and repression, thereby preventing id or primary process material from gaining access to consciousness.

COUNTERCONDITIONING Utilized in behavior therapy techniques, this is a process of producing a different response to an identical stimulus not harmonious with the original response to which the person was already conditioned.

COUNTERDEPENDENT Refers to individuals who will do anything to prevent the development of any dependent relationship.

COUNTERPHOBIC A flight toward the content of the phobia rather than the flight away from it. It is an attempt at mastery through denial and impulsive preemptory behavior.

COUNTERTRANSFERENCE The psychoanalyst's unconscious reactions to the patient that ultimately should be understood by the analyst. The key here is that conscious reactions toward the patient—either positive or negative—are considered the analyst's transference to the patient. Such conscious reactions can usually be more readily managed by the analyst. It is the countertransferential feelings and rather oblique identification with negative aspects of the patient's behavior and attitudes that interferes with the analyst's perception, understanding, and interventions and can at times be understood as the analyst's projective identification. Thus, in order to have a better grip on the therapeutic process, the analyst needs to make such unconscious self material more available, more conscious. Elimination of the countertransferential interference presumably enables the analyst to retain a more objective stance in the absence of personal interfering material. Contributors to the study of countertransference include Bion, Gill, Grinberg, Lang, R. Marshall, S. Marshall, Racker, Sandler, Searles, Winnicott, E. Wolfe, and Wolstein. See Projective identification; Transference.

CROSS-DRESSING Usually considered synonymous with transvestism. Essentially referring to donning clothing of the opposite sex so that a feeling of well-being or sexually tinged gratification results, or both.

CROSS-GENDER DISORDER Desire to acquire the attributes of the opposite sex in a variety of ways without necessarily feeling obsessed about wanting to change sex—as in transsexuality.

CROWDING, THOUGHT Schizophrenic patients often complain of feeling that their thoughts are crowded. This generally means that the person feels overwhelmed or overcome by too many thoughts, where the plethora of thoughts begin to occupy space in the mind designed for fewer thoughts as well as "having time" for those thoughts that are paced more slowly.

CUNNILINGUS Oral sex performed on a female.

CURATIVE FACTORS MODEL Formulated by Yalom to identify those variables that promote growth in therapy groups.

CUTTING Referred to as self-mutilation. Cutting takes place on all parts of the body (usually with a razor blade). The cutting is most often superficial, although blood is drawn. Legs, arms, wrist, hips, and breasts are frequent bodily locations of the cutting. It is mostly seen in women who report a relief of tension after the cutting is completed. See Self; Self-mutilation.

CYCLOTHYMIA Milder form of manic-depression.

D

DANTO, ELIZABETH ANN (1952). Author, *Freud's Free Clinics—Psychoanalysis and Social Justice, 1918–1938.* Associate professor, Hunter College School of Social Work, City University of New York. Former commissioner on employment and economic support for the National Association of social workers. Member, editorial board, *Dictionary of Psychopathology.*

DAYDREAM Conscious fantasy usually of a compensatory nature that satisfies some wish, and, in this sense, daydreaming generally relieves tension, insecurities, and inadequacy feelings. Daydreams also can become acts of withdrawal in which revenge or sexual themes are expressed, although not usually acted out. Hence, the expression "You can't go to jail for what you're thinking." All people experience daydreams; in the normal sense they represent a person's stepping "behind the line"—so to speak—to take a breath and then return to an in "front of the line" position in the real world. See Line, The.

DAY'S RESIDUE Elements of the day's events preceding a dream that become incorporated in the dream. In psychoanalytic dream work, seen to contain a pivotal element motivating the dream.

DEATH INSTINCT This proposed instinct most often presents itself as an aggressive impulse. In contrast, with the life instinct, known as eros, and representing libidinal energy supporting attachment to objects, the death instinct, known as thanatos and reflecting the death instinct energy called destrudo is ultimately turned inward, serving the goal of death. Destrudo energy reflects the instinct toward eternal rest. It essentially means the wish to reduce one's tension index to zero, thereby satisfying the derivative wish of the pleasure principle—for full pleasure, satisfaction of wishes, and absence of tension.

DECOMPENSATION The undoing of defense mechanisms. Thus, with respect to decompensation, a breakdown or a return to more primitive functioning is seen, as in schizophrenic behavior and / or thinking.

DECONDITIONING See Desensitization, systematic.

DEDIFFERENTIATION A regressive state of the psychological organization of the person, usually applied in the diagnosis of schizophrenia in children.

DEEP COGNITIONS In cognitive behavior therapy, these are core beliefs (schemas).

DEFENSE Usually applied to ego function, the purpose of which is to protect the person from their own impulses and tensions. Contributors to the literature on defenses include Bond, Buckley, Burry, Dahl, Drake, A. Freud, Greenwald, Grotstein, Reich, Valliant, Wallerstein.

DEFENSE MECHANISMS Specific defenses attributed to ego function that are designed also to guard against anxiety by managing specific emotions. For example, displacement frequently is used to manage anger, among other uses and functions—as, for example, in dreams, or compensation, which is frequently used to counteract depression.

Compartmentalization—reduces anxiety by keeping aspects of personality apart.

Compensation—designed to elevate mood and avoid inferiority feelings.

Denial—utilized in order not to "see" something.

Displacement—utilized to direct anger to less threatening figures. See Displacement

Identification—enables the consolidation of one's persona.
Intellectualization—using logic, rather than emotion.
Internalization—imprinting of values.
Introjection—built on the foundation of identification, but more differentiated.
Isolation—separation of intellect and emotion.
Projection—attributing unfavorable qualities to another that the subject is unwilling to admit about the self.
Projective identification—attributing part of the self to the other, which is then repudiated (if you spot it, you got it), and identifying with it.
Rationalization—justification for any behavior.
Reaction-formation—turn into the opposite as a function of attraction.
Regression—receding to more immature functioning.
Repression—sinking into the unconscious.
Splitting—separating good and bad qualities in the object.
Sublimation—goal-oriented activity instead of focus on impulses.
Symbolization—disguising ideas and feelings.
Turning against the self—making hostility more tolerable by directing it to the self.
Undoing—taking back the decision or commitment—undoing it.

DÉJÀ VU A momentary feeling by which a person could swear that the exact presently occurring circumstance happened in the past. It has been reported that in some cases, during the déjà vu, the person can predict what will happen in the ensuing moment or two before the situation ends. Analagous to a hypnagogic hallucination.

DELERIUM, EMOTIONAL An experience in which a person believes in a false idea and then behaves accordingly.

DELERIUM, IDIOPATHIC A psychiatric condition usually caused by brain injury.

DELUSION A false belief that is elaborated and rationalized in the face of even blatant evidence to the contrary. Such delusions are usually seen in paranoid schizophrenic people, although encapsulated delusions can also be nonpsychotic symptoms of the defense of turning against the self, basically as a way to contain hostility. Delusions of persecution consist of the person's certainty that various outside forces have harmful intentions. This is usually understood as the person's own superego force exerting itself as a guilty conscience and then projecting such intentions onto objects in the environment. Frequently this sort of persecutory delusion is represented by the person's sense that being led into sin or some other delinquent behavior is generated by the mandate of the delusion. Another major delusional category is the grandiose delusion. In grandiose delusions the person expresses thoughts that can be considered megalomaniacal, or omnipotent, both of which are rationalized as based upon pure altruism. In such delusions the person feels that some special privilege—usually from God—has been granted. Both delusional categories—persecutory and grandiose—are described as delusions of reference where everything that occurs is a reference to the self. Delusions of reference are the quintessential solipsistic projections.

DELUSION, ENCAPSULATED Usually referred to in paranoid schizophrenic states in which a delusion is presumably entirely isolated from the overall personality so that the pathology of the delusion is relegated solely to its delusional perimeter. Thus the delusion is encapsulated and not necessarily contaminating the remainder of the personality.

DELUSION, PERSECUTORY See Delusion.

DELUSIONAL DISORDER Characterized by the presence of conventional delusions.

DELUSIONAL PERCEPTION Attributing extra meaning to standard stimuli as a result of distorted thinking. Seen as a precursor to a full flowering of a psychotic delusion.

DEMANDINGNESS (DEM) In rational emotive behavior therapy, demands for perfection, comfort, control, and certainty are considered to be the foundation of most human disturbance, both emotional and behavioral, leading, in turn, to awfulizing, low frustration tolerance, and negative self and other rating.

DEMENTIA A condition in which the person's cognitive, intellectual, and personality functioning continuously erodes so that the person becomes, for all intents and purposes, non compos mentis.

DEMENTIA PRAECOX Arcane diagnosis related to psychoses in which the prognosis is guarded, deterioration of the personality is evident, and remission is no longer a possibility. See Kraepelin, Emil.

DEMONIC POSSESSION Considered by believers to be an evil spirit that gains control of one's body and psyche.

DENIAL A defense mechanism attributed to ego function in which the person tends not to see or acknowledge information that is distasteful. This is considered a major defense of the hysteric personality, who tends to see that which feels good and avoids seeing anything that might cause tension. Equivalent to selective perception and perceptual defense. See Anosognosia; Defense mechanisms.

DEPENDENCY A personality characteristic and/or need reflecting the person's reliance on a nurturing and/or authority figure.

DEPENDENCY GROUP See Assumption group.

DEPERSONALIZATION A condition that is frequently considered in existential terms as a feeling or condition of differentness. The person feels strangely different—other than the usual self. In the schizophrenic condition the depersonalized state can be sustained for long periods. Under nonschizophrenic conditions depersonalization can disappear as suddenly as it originally appeared. It is also referred to as a feeling of derealization.

DEPERSONALIZATION DISORDER In *DSM* nomenclature a condition in which the person feels generally detached, strange, and different.

DEPRESSION Referred to as a diagnostic category. Characterized by a anhedoniclike state, with constituent factors of loss of interest, moodiness, psychomotor retardation, absence of motivation, fatigue, infrequency of bathing, cognitive difficulty (usually with respect to concentration as well as attention span), suicidal thoughts, sleep problems such as insomnia, lessening of sexual interest, loss of appetite, and any number of other such symptoms that can represent a withdrawal from the person's typical and normal activity. In depression the emotion of sorrow or sadness is accompanied by feelings of pessimism. Psychoanalytically, depression is also understood to imply repression of anger. In neuropsychoanalysis depression may be characterized by altered activities of the neuromodulators dopamine, noradrenaline, and serotonin.

DEPRESSION, AGITATED In this sort of depression the person is visibly irritable and impatient; an increase in psychomotor activity also becomes apparent.

DEPRESSION, ANACLITIC See Anaclitic depression.

DEPRESSION, *DSM* DIAGNOSES In the *Diagnostic and Statistical Manual* of the American Psychiatric Association depression has been parsed in the following ways:

Depression, endogenous—A result of constitutional factors.

Depression, exogenous—A result of a distressing event.

Depression, involutional—Used synonymously with involutional psychosis or involutional melancholia. Refers to women, ages forty to fifty-five, and to men, ages fifty to sixty-five, who exhibit a syndrome of a focus on delusion, obsession, and digestion. The delusional material usually consists of guilt, the obsession is with death, and a digestive preoccupation is with anything concerning the gastrointestinal tract. Those who develop this disorder usually have no prior history of hospitalization for any mental illness. Paranoid ideation is seen, and it is thought that the involutional despair is a function of a sense that life has passed such a person by and that such a person is no longer useful in the ways that had previously offered a sense of importance.

Depression, postpartum—Depression seen in women immediately after giving birth.

Depression, unipolar—See Unipolar.

Depressive, major disorder—presence of major depression—the severest form of depression.

DEPRESSION, REACTIVE A depression triggered by a recent event that, because of its acute nature, has a good prognosis. The purpose of the reactive depression is to allay anxiety. This particular diagnosis is no longer officially designated in the latest *DSM* nosology, although it remains clinically useful.

DEPRESSIVE POSITION See Klein, Melanie.

DEREALIZATION Similar to depersonalization. The person feels alien to immediate surroundings as though things are not quite real—in a sense, derealized. It is an experience frequently reported by schizophrenic patients.

DEREFLECTION In logotherapy this is antithetical to excessive attention on symptoms, rather concerning a focus on interpersonal productive interaction. See Logotherapy.

DERIVATIVE BEHAVIOR Behavior that is derived, or an eventual sample of behavior, representing some original source out of which the behavior stems. For example, in psychoanalytic understanding, feelings of dependency would be considered derivative of the oral level of psychosexual conflict.

DESENSITIZATION, SYSTEMATIC See Systematic desensitization.

DESEXUALIZATION The person's energy, associated with libido, impulse, and primary process, is diverted instead to ego functions and secondary process.

DESTRUDO Refers to the psychoanalytic construct of the death instinct. See Death instinct.

DETERIORATION INDEX A measure of intellectual or cognitive impairment on the Wechsler-Bellevue Intelligence Scales based upon a comparison of those subtests showing strong decline with those that are not so impaired.

DETERMINISM The philosophical position that derivative products can be traced to original cause and effect events. Psychoanalysis is deterministic.

DEUTSCH, HELENE (1884–1982). European-born American psychoanalyst. First woman in Freud's inner circle. Contributed to the understanding of narcissism, focused on the psychology of women, and was generally known as a psychoanalyst extraordinaire. See As-if personality.

DEVELOPMENTAL DISORDERS Referring to childhood disorders concerning either disorders of arrested development, functional learning disorders, or those of biological origins.

Developmental disorders, pervasive—autism as well as the variety of autistic syndromes are considered pervasive developmental disorders characterized by pathological or arrested development of language and overall social behavior.

Developmental disorders, specific—these are disorders of language, academic skills, and motor skills.

DEVELOPMENTAL INVARIANCE Seen in cases of arrested development in which, as the child ages chronologically, there is no corresponding change, for example, in age-appropriate speech development.

DEVELOPMENTAL LEVELS Chronological age separated by stages of development from infancy to older age. Essentially, the divisions of stages begin with the neonatal period to the infancy stage to early childhood, mid-childhood, preadolescence, adolescence, adulthood, and finally older age.

DEVELOPMENTAL NEUROPSYCHOLOGY Relating brain and behavior in child development with respect to cognitive abilities, disturbances of personality such as schizophrenia, and language problems like those that appear with aphasia.

DEVELOPMENTAL PSYCHOLOGY The aspect of psychology designed to focus on the normative levels of child development in all respects: cognitive, intellectual, emotional, social. Jean Piaget, (1896–1980), a Swiss psychologist, was particularly influential in the study of such normative levels. Child and adolescent psychotherapy focuses on the behavior and emotional life of those children who demonstrate a wide variety of acting out behaviors reflecting emotional imbalance, psychological maladjustment, and the consequences of family pathology. An example of this specialty in treatment and research with children, adolescents, and parents, is the work of Anni Bergman and of A. E. Kazdin of the Yale Child Study Center, president of the American Psychological Association.

DIAGNOSIS Deriving the salient abstraction out of an entire syndrome of symptoms and labeling it. Deriving parsimony from a universe of pathology.

DIALECTICAL BEHAVIORAL THERAPY (DBT). A therapy developed by American psychologist Marcia Linehan combining cognitive behavior therapy with that of Eastern Zen practice. Initially utilized with borderline personality disorders, it is also reputed to be helplful with depressive, anxious, suicidal, addictive, and other resistant and emotionally labile clients. Promotes "wisemind," a state between a rational and more emotional state of mind. The four aims of DBT:

1. *mindfulness*—skills of *what* to do and *how* to do it;
2. *interpersonal effectiveness*—a learning trajectory in the increased likelihood of meeting goals;
3. *distress tolerance*—learning to tolerate stress;
4. *emotional regulation*—self-soothing of emotional upset through the use of meditation.

See Linehan, Marcia.

DIMS (DISORDERS OF INITIATING AND MAINTAINING SLEEP) Referring to insomnia. See Sleep Disorders.

DIRECT ANALYSIS A form of therapy developed by Rosen in which the therapist will play the part of the parent with a measured disregard of conventional therapeutic boundaries. Designed for use with psychotic individuals, but not an accepted form of therapy within mainstream professional work.

DISEASE, FLIGHT INTO This is an attempt to escape from the tensions and challenges of everyday life by retreating into some dysfunctional state. It can be considered the science of achieving secondary gain—that is, protection, care, nurturance, and pity. See Gain, secondary.

DISOWNING PROJECTION In the relational psychologies, as, for example, in intersubjectivity theory, disowning projection is the attribution of personal hated faults (unconscious though they may be) to the object group.

DISPLACEMENT Transferring emotion or ideas to another object. Displacement is a dream work mechanism in Freudian dream analysis. Displacement of affect is frequently seen in schizophrenic patients. It is also considered to be one of the ego-defense mechanisms.

DISPUTING In rational emotive behavior therapy, considered to be the confrontation of beliefs individuals hold about themselves and the world that are essentially invalid or at least unsubstantiated. Also referred to as disputation.

DISSOCIATION Usually can be understood as a parsing of the mental life so that the person behaves in ways that are automatic and not particularly of an observing-ego position. Dissociation is seen in fugues, schizophrenia, and in multiple or dissociated identity disordered individuals (formerly known as split or multiple personality).

DISSOCIATIVE DISORDERS Those that are considered disorders of identity and contain symptoms expressed in a variety of forms.

Amnesia—in which memory is lost for any number of events or eras of the person's life.

Conversion hysteria—in which symbolic expression of tension appears as a physical or sensory manifestation of the tension.

Dissociative identity disorder—probably the most fascinating of the dissociative disorders. Its most popular form has been referred to as split personality and it was originally considered demon possession, after which it came to be known as alter personality. With the onset of *DSM* classification systems, it has been called split personality. In the latter part of the twentieth century it morphed into the designation *multiple personality,* and its most recent incarnation is *dissociative identity disorder.* Essentially, the formation of personality in this disorder has a basic tripartate structure.

The host personality—this is the person's consciousness of the self. However, such a person is not conscious of the other two personalities inhabiting the psyche—the aggressive and the sexual.

The aggressive personality—a personality solely devoted to expressing anger and aggression. Is aware of the presence of the host as well as the presence of the sexual personality.

The sexual personality—a personality devoted solely to sexual behavior such as seduction, exhibitionism, and other sexual preoccupations. Is aware of the presence of the host as well as the presence of the aggressive personality.

Psychoanalytically, it is thought that because of a traumatically ongoing prohibition against acknowledging one's anger and sexuality, the person then separates these aspects of emotion so that a guilt-free consciousness regarding their presence can exist: hence three personalities in one person—host, aggressive, and sexual. Etiology is thought to be characterized by abuse, physical, sexual, or a combination of the two.

Fugue states—reflecting an interruption of conscious awareness.
Multiple personality—See Dissociative Identity Disorder.
Schizophrenia—in an overarching sense with respect to the appearance of delusions and hallucinations.

DISTORTION Referring to perception and used as a central concept in psychoanalytic treatment insofar as the interpretation of transference is said to be effective in creating a corrective experience for the patient regarding such distortions. This corrective experience is, for the most part, the correction of distortions that were the basis of the patient's attitudes, anxieties, and dissatisfactions.

DISTORTION, EGO See Ego distortion.

DISTORTION, PARATAXIC Referring to a distorted identification based upon a transferential response.

DOES (DISORDERS OF EXCESSIVE SOMNOLENCE) See Sleep disorders.

DOPAMINERGIC "SEEKING" SYSTEM According to Panksepp in the domain of neuropsychoanlysis, this system corresponds to Freud's concept of libido. See Panksepp, Jaak.

DOPPELGANGER The rather idiosyncratic notion that somewhere every person has a double. In delusional states the person is convinced of the presence of such a person.

DORA One of Freud's classic cases published in the early part of the twentieth century and titled *Fragment of an Analysis of a Case of Hysteria.* The case enabled Freud to elaborate and relate his theory of dreams and symptoms to the vicissitudes and repression of sexual impulses. The ostensible causative gist of Dora's concern was that she was barter for the husband whose wife was having an affair with her father. Of course, given Freud's theory of sexual repression and symptoms, he rather overlooked the conflict Dora may have had between some erotic engagement, on the one hand, and, on the other, her probable anger (or perhaps rage) at her father for the ostensible trade-off. In addition, the shame of being the oedipal loser (the unfavorite) and, to boot, with someone who was not even her mother perhaps corresponds to Dora's identification with her mother, and, therefore, it could be imagined that Dora's anger was quite likely directed to the intruder-woman as well—and for more than one reason. Thus, hypothetically, the emotional culprit in the hysterical reaction may have been anger rather than sex.

DOUBLE BIND A concept developed by Bateson and applied to schizophrenic psychodynamics. It is proposed that the schizophrenic person received simultaneous contradictory messages from the parent and as a result could not process thoughts logically.

DOWN SYNDROME Brain birth defect presenting distorted bodily features. Formerly referred to in the professional as well as popular lexicon as Mongolism.

DOWNWARD ARROW TECHNIQUE In cognitive behavior therapy this is used to locate and identify dysfunctional beliefs in order for them to crystallize in a more conscious form.

DREAM Interest in dream research became significantly more common in the latter part of the twentieth century. Research has revealed that all individuals dream and that dreams occur approximately every ninety minutes—each dream emerging up from deep sleep or stage 4 sleep to lighter stages of sleep. Thus sleeping for about seven or so hours yields four to five dreams. See REM (Rapid Eye Movement).

DREAM THEORY, FREUDIAN Freud reasoned that the dream helps keep the dreamer sleeping because the raw material of the dream—its latent content—is too upsetting and would typically awaken the dreamer. Because the latent dream (referred to as "the dream from below") is translated into its manifest version (the descriptive dream story that is remembered and referred to as "the dream from above"), it will not likely disturb sleep to the extent of awakening the dreamer so disguised and unthreatening. Thus, according to Freud, a prime (although not sole) function of the dream is to guard sleep. Freud also proposed that all dreams are wish fulfillments. The following are key concepts of Freudian dream theory.

Dream, anxiety—a dream that is disturbing, although not on the level of the nightmare. The anxiety dream is usually one in which the dreamer, although in a state of discomfort, nevertheless remains asleep. The nightmare, on the other hand, is defined as always awakening the dreamer.

Dream day residue—that part of the previous day's event that insinuates itself into the dream material.

Dream determinant—referring to an element of the dream that may be used for free association. Its past use referred rather exclusively to the pivotal theme or stimulus for the dream's occurrence in the first place, and this dream determinant was seen as the key point of the patient's dynamic.

Dream function—in addition to the function of the dream as a guardian of sleep, Freud suggested that the function of the dream was to express the patient's wish; thus every dream contains a major wish that informs the dream and around which the dream revolves.

Dream, latent—the underlying raw material of the dream that is translated into the manifest story line of the dream. In psychoanalytic treatment it is the latent meaning(s) of the dream that aims to be uncovered.

Dream, manifest—the story line of the dream. Freud discovered (or postulated) that the manifest dream becomes realized out of the latent underlying raw material of the dream, through the dream mechanisms of

- *condensation*—objects or ideas can be compressed.
- *displacement*—an emotion can be transferred to another person.
- *secondary elaboration*—the dream can be stitched together by a series of interstitial connections so that it

makes some sense as a logical, or nearly logical, story; such connections are identified as elaborations. Secondary elaboration works on the latent material of the dream in an attempt to translate this latent, more threatening material into the manifest less threatening dream.

- *symbolization*—one thing can be a symbol for another.

Dream, nightmare—defined as dream content that always awakens the dreamer. See Nightmare.

Dream, overdetermination—See Overdetermination.

Dream stimulus—either internal or external pivotal event that sets off the dream.

Other than Freud, a sample of the many theorists of dreams and their function include Altman, Bonime, Empson, Gutheil, Hartmann, R. M. Jones, Kellerman, and E. F. Sharpe.

DREAM WORK MECHANISMS Freudian postulates regarding how the dream forms its story line, known as the manifest level of the dream. These mechanisms include condensation, displacement, secondary elaboration, and symbolization. See Dream theory, Freudian.

DRIVE In the mental apparatus this is the psychological-biological energy that strives for expression, thereby creating tension that psychological behavior is designed to relieve. Considered to be biologically given, Freud postulated the drives of life and death, which have come to be accepted as the sexual and aggressive drives. In neuropsychoanalytic understanding, drives are seen as a series of basic emotions—motives to action—that are based in the pontine brain regions. These emotions include play, exploration, fear, anger, sorrow, caring—all related to a Freudian dynamic unconscious.

DSM DIAGNOSTIC AND STATISTICAL MANUAL OF MENTAL DISORDERS This is the official diagnostic tool of the American Psychiatric Association. In the past fifty years it has gone through five revisions, with the sixth in progress. Contributors associated with the construction of modern *DSM* nomenclatures include Alan Frances and Robert L. Spitzer. A multiaxial system is employed, and, of the five axes in the DSM architecture, Axes I and II refer to diagnostic entities. Diagnostic entities are defined by the presence of observable symptoms or behaviors, eschewing theoretical bias. See Sydenham, Thomas.

DUAL ASPECT MONISM See Neuropsychoanalysis.

DUAL INSTINCT THEORY Freud suggested instincts of two antagonistic types. These were the ego instincts and sexual instincts. Later, they were categorized as life and death instincts, also known as eros and thanatos or aggression and sex. The antagonism of the instincts was perceived as the basis for conflict.

DYING, STAGES OF Five stages proposed by E. Kubler-Ross: 1. denial, 2. anger, 3. bargaining, 4. depression, 5. resignation and detachment.

DYNAMIC The interaction of underlying attitudes, transferences, moods, and tensions that comprise the personality configuration of any individual.

DYSFUNCTIONAL NEGATIVE FEELINGS In cognitive behavior therapy this is a reference to disturbed feelings such as anxiety, hostility, depression, guilt or shame that keep people from achieving their goals. In contrast, functional negative feelings refers to such feelings as sadness, regret, disappointment, or apprehension—emotions that allow people to be motivated to continue to pursue their goals.

DYSKINESIA, TARDIVE See Tardive dyskinesia.

DYSLEXIA Seen in children who have difficulty reading and spelling and considered to be a developmental disorder. Words, numbers, or letters can be seen backwards or as being unstable on the page. Considered to be a genetic anomaly.

DYSMORPHIA The delusion or false belief that some defect characterizes the person's body.

Dysmorphia, somatoform type—obsession with some imagined defect, although not reaching the level of delusion.

Dysmorphophobia—serious dysmorphia in which the patient creates all functioning and life's plans around the dysmorphic concern. Can be reflective of a psychosis.

DYSPHORIA Unhappiness and pessimism.

DYSSOMNIA Sleep disorder. The dyssomnias include

primary insomnia—difficulty in initiating and maintaining sleep;

primary hypersomnia—excessive sleepiness;

breathing-related sleep disorder—such as in an apnea syndrome;

circadian rhythm sleep disorder—sleep-wake schedule problem.

See Narcolepsy; Parasomnia; Sleep apnea; Sleep disorders.

DYSTHYMIA A contemporary formulation for depressive conditions in which individuals feel dejected, sad, hopeless, and pessimistic. Suicidal ideation can also be present and self-esteem typically becomes depleted.

DYSTONIC Referring to feeling out of sorts. In psychoanalytic usage, dystonic refers to a condition in which anxiety is experienced. This becomes synonymous with the ego-alien, in contrast to the syntonic, which refers to a condition in which the person does not experience anxiety and, indeed, feels in sync with typical personality patterns of the self.

E

EARLY MEMORY See Memory, early.

ECLECTICISM Referring to practitioners who are not committed to any one approach. They will utilize whatever approach appears likely to work with patients, while drawing technique, interpretation, and understanding from a wide spectrum of theories and treatment modalities.

ECO-MAP An ecology map that identifies pertinent individuals, groups, and larger systems of the subject's life. It is a graphic representation, with the subject in the center of a circle and influential variables including social institutions—family, school—and environmental influences surrounding the center.

ECONOMIC THEORY In psychoanalysis, refers to the distribution of instinctual energy, such as libido. See Freud, Sigmund.

ECTOMORPH See Sheldon, William Herbert.

EGO In psychoanalytic theory, the ego is conceived to be part of the tripartite structural psychic apparatus of id, superego, and ego. It is that part of the psychic apparatus that mediates between the inner urges, on the one hand, and the demands of reality, on the other, and is governed entirely by the secondary process—that which assures the individual adequate reality testing, frustration tolerance, and realistic judgment. The ego is also considered to be that part of the psychic organization that generates and calibrates mechanisms of defense designed to manage anxiety.

EGO, BODY The body ego refers to the amalgam of ideas and feelings about one's body, with regard to one's self-perception, or with respect to one's ego—all more or less synonymous.

EGO, SURFACE See Surface ego.

EGO-ALIEN Stimuli unacceptable to the ego are considered ego-alien or ego-dystonic. Stimuli that are dystonic or alien generate anxiety, unlike stimuli that are ego-syntonic (opposite of dystonic), which cause no anxiety.

EGO BOUNDARY A topographical concept of the boundary of abstraction, distinguishing between inner signals and impulses in contrast to environmental or external demands of reality.

EGO DISTORTION Frequently seen in relation to discussions of the ego's function as the container for the operation of defense mechanisms. Such distortion would reflect an impairment of the ego's ability to utilize mechanisms of defense to best advantage.

EGO DRIVE Drive for self-preservation in Freud's earliest conception of instinct theory, which included a libidinal or broad sexual drive as well.

EGO-DYSTONIC Stimuli unacceptable to the conscious self and to the ego. Wishes that are incompatible with a person's ideals and therefore those that generate anxiety. See Ego-alien.

EGO FRAGMENTATION Refers to a decompensation process in which the person begins to express pathological symptoms.

EGO FUNCTION In psychoanalysis, ego function is related to secondary process and reality testing. The ego is the agency that interprets the external world and drives other functions such as awareness of self, memory, motor activity, problem solving, and management of impulses.

EGO IDEAL The condition in which a person will identify with an admired figure and then use that identified image as a guide for one's own attitudes and behavior. These ego-ideal figures are considered to be post-parental figures.

EGO IDENTITY See Kernberg, Otto.

EGO PSYCHOLOGY An ego psychology perspective holds that the ego has its own energy—different from instinctual wishes. The focus is on adaptation in relation to interpersonal and cultural variables, thus away from psychoanalytic drive theory. Essentially it is the arena of dynamic psychology in which the focus is on internalization of parental imperatives known as parental introjects. The importance of the internalization and introjection process also implies the importance of the influence of external forces in the environment and, in a larger sense, the influence of culture. A sample of ego psychologists as well as those theoreticians interested in the nature of ego include Blanck, G., Blanck, R., Hartmann, Kriss, Lowenstein, and Menaker, all of whom focused on a sharper definition of the self other than that embraced by "ego."

EGO RESISTANCE See Resistance, ego.

EGO STRENGTH The relative resilience of the ego with respect to its ability to manage the pressures of the environment, the pressures of the id, as well as that of the superego. Includes ability to tolerate frustration and the ability to postpone immediate needs for gratification.

EGO-SYNTONIC Stimuli that are acceptable to the ego so that anxiety is not generated, unlike ego-alien or ego-dystonic stimuli, which generate anxiety. See Ego-alien.

EGOCENTRISM Roughly equivalent to solipsistic functioning, or a narcissistic orientation, in which everything is known through one's needs, impulses, and wishes, with little or no input from independent sources.

EGOISM Refers to one's greediness and selfishness, in contrast to the term *egotism*, which refers to a prevailing sense of self-importance and even grandiosity.

EGOTISM One's focus on self-aggrandizement. See Egoism.

EIDETIC IMAGERY Referring to especially vivid memory of written material. Usually appearing in childhood, but in most cases disappearing with maturity. The person's memory is characterized by unusual clarity and precision. Evidence exists that this type of memory is biochemically determined, which accounts for its difference from the more typical kind of memory.

ELASTICITY PRINCIPLE Ferenczi's notion of flexibility in the analyst's approach to the patient. See Ferenczi, Sandor.

ELECTRA COMPLEX A Jungian construct that is for all intents and purposes equivalent on the female side to the oedipal conflict. See Oedipus complex.

ELECTROCONVULSIVE THERAPY (ECT) Referred to as electroshock therapy. Electrodes on the scalp send an electric current through the brain. The patient then experiences a seizure. Used frequently in mental hospitals and especially applied (with decent success) to severely depressed patients.

ELECTROENCEPHALOGRAM (EEG) Recorded electrical activity of the brain.

ELECTROSHOCK THERAPY See Electroconvulsive therapy.

ELEGANT REBT (RATIONAL EMOTIVE BEHAVIOR THERAPY) Based on the belief that disputing only clients' inferences or attributions is superficial, since it leaves the deeper philosophic assumptions underlying them untouched. Elegant disputing, challenging shoulds, awfulizing, frustration intolerance, and global self or other rating are seen as necessary for profound attitudinal change—getting better as opposed to merely feeling better. See Inelegant REBT.

ELLIS, ALBERT (1913–2007). Pioneering American psychologist who, in 1956, and after becoming dissatisfied with psychoanalysis, introduced the first of the cognitive behavior therapies, rational emotive behavior therapy (REBT). Considered a humanistic approach by Ellis and deriving from his immersion in philosophy, REBT's premise is that people are not disturbed by things, but by the views they take of them. Although many dysfunctional beliefs may have been acquired in childhood, they continue to be reinforced in adulthood through a process of self-indoctrination and can be changed through a process of logical and functional disputation, without the necessity of an archaeological excavation of one's past. Ellis is arguably now more influential than Freud in changing the face of psychotherapy with over two thirds of American psychologists currently identifying themselves as practicing some form of cognitive behavior therapy. Psychoanalysis is now better represented, correspondingly, in the curricula of the humanities and general social sciences. Luminaries associated with the Albert Ellis Institute have included David Burns, Cyril Franks, Arnold Lazarus, Paul Meehl, Penelope Russianoff, and Janet L. Wolfe. See REBT.

ELLIS, H. HAVELOCK (1859–1939). British psychologist known for early research on issues of sex.

EMOTION Emotions are generally accepted as evolved transitory states designed to manage adaptational challenges. Mood is a more sustained state. Emotion contains experienced, behavioral, and physiological components. In the broad sweep of theory and research on emotion, three traditions emerge. The first concerns the evolutionary or psychoevolutionary tradition as seen in the theories and work of Plutchik, Scott, and Eibl-Eibesfeldt. The second tradition is the psychophysiological context as seen in the theories and work of Tomkins, Izard, Lazarus, Mandler, and Pribram, and including Schachter and Singer with respect to cognitive arousal theory. The third tradition is the psychodynamic one, as seen in the theories and work of Brenner, Averill, and Spezzano. With respect to psychotherapy treatment, the psychodynamic and cognitive behavior therapy orientations, along with a variety of other therapy modalities, claim special knowledge with respect to having therapeutic entrée to the emotions and their vicissitudes. Several theories of emotion agree on the presence of only a few primary emotions that combine in various ways (and with respect to their intensities—e.g., annoyance, anger, rage) to form all the thousands of complex or secondary states. The primary emotions that find themselves on the primary emotion lists of most theorists include acceptance, disgust, fear, anger, joy, and sorrow, with expectation, surprise, love, shame, happiness, shyness, and hate also appearing on various lists. As examples of additional interest in the study of emotion—especially in the concern with identifying basic emotions—Cattell derived ten factors of basic emotions and Darwin listed seven clusters of emotion. According to LeDoux, and in the domain of neuropsychoanalysis, the memory of an emotion is considered to be the cool memory, while emotional memory is called the hot memory. According to neuroscientist Schore, the right hemisphere of the brain is considered the locus of the emotional brain. See Drive; Limbic system; Pontine regions.

EMOTIONAL INTELLIGENCE Concerns variations of social intelligence, native intelligence, and variations of frames of mind. Contributors include Howard Gardner and Daniel Goleman.

EMOTIONAL REASONING In cognitive behavioral therapy, a form of cognitive distortion in which people assume that their negative emotions reflect the way things really are: "I feel (worthless), therefore it must be true." In contrast, in neuropsychoanalytic understanding such a definition overvalues reason over emotion. In uncertain contexts, right brain intuitive processes are more adaptive than left brain reason. A reduced capacity for emotional learning and an overreliance on analytic secondary process cognition is then also maladaptive.

EMOTION LEARNING A concept utilized in neuropsychoanalysis. During times of uncertainty decisions are likely to be made on the basis of emotion or intuition. Such learning or decision making becomes impaired in persons with lesions to the frontal lobes, and such individuals will generally tend to make poor choices, even though they may possess good intelligence.

EMOTIVE TECHNIQUES. Various techniques that are vigorous, vivid, and dramatic. Used in REBT, cognitive behavior therapy, and some experiential approaches to help people get in better touch with their feelings, improve expression of their feelings, and move from intellectual insight to emotional insight.

EMPATHY Imagining oneself into the subjective experience of another person. Putting oneself in another's shoes can reveal what that person is feeling. The ability to empathize is one of the therapeutic contributions that advances the treatment. It can be the key to deepening the treatment by providing the therapist with a broader grasp of transferential as well as countertransferential material. Empathy is also the cornerstone of Kohutian self-psychology and has influenced the development of intersubjective theory as well as playing a part in other psychodynamic orientations. Empathy is also a cornerstone of a Rogerian construct regarding the therapist's view of the client. See Rogers, Carl.

EMPIRICISM Basing one's sense of the world on experience rather than on theory or statistics. "It's an empirical question," essentially means, "Let's wait and see how it turns out."

ENACTMENT In the relational psychotherapeutic orientation, enactment refers to the relationship between patient and analyst, who are considered to be in an inevitable unconscious collusion, the mutuality of which is thought to reflect unconscious fantasy.

ENCAPSULATED DELUSION See Delusion, encapsulated.

ENCOPRESIS Rather than based upon voluntary bowel movement, defecation is the result of psychopathology—as in acting out—or of some developmental arrest or mental retardation. The problem is not biologically or genetically based. Also referred to as elimination disorder, where feces are deposited in inappropriate places (clothing).

ENDOGENOUS Clinical conditions, the source of which are biological, and not a result of environmental stimuli.

Contrasts with exogenous. See Depression; DSM diagnoses; Exogenous.

ENDOMORPH See Sheldon, William Herbert.

ENDOPSYCHIC STRUCTURE Uncertain sense of self, with ego weakness correlated to early parental (maternal) underachievement in relation to the child. Formulated by Fairbairn and further developed by Guntrip.

ENGULFMENT See Enmeshment.

ENMESHMENT Refers to the overinvolvement of one family member with another or of one partner of a relationship with the other. The overinvolvement is considered to be of a pathological nature and is essentially emotionally and psychologically disabling, which results in a significant compromise of interpersonal functioning.

ENOSIOPHOBIA The conviction one has of being guilty of some profoundly immoral or unlawful act. See Pseudomania.

ENTROPY In psychoanalytic parlance, referring to a loss of powers with age.

ENURESIS Bedwetting.

EPIDEMIOLOGY Study of the incidence of diseases as well as the variety of factors associated with the appearance of diseases.

EPIGENESIS Phenomena that apply to human psychological development concern genetic givens that, in order to materialize, await their environmental salience—they need a relevant environmental stimulus or stimuli as the ignition to the phenomenon's appearance. Thus certain behaviors, for example, can be said to have an epigenetic underpinning.

EPILEPSY A convulsive state that is organically based. General types are

Grand mal state—a major convulsion takes place with full body spasms, seizures, and convulsions, frequently followed by disorientation, long periods of sleep, and some amnesia for the event. The sensation of auras is typical.

Petit mal state—the person is dazed, and the disturbance is briefer and milder than that of the grand mal state.

Flicker fusion—an epileptic seizure caused by flickering visual stimulation.

EPILEPTIC CRY This is the crying or gasping sound of the epileptic person at the beginning of the epileptic episode.

EPINOSIC GAIN A secondary gain, as in the appearance of a psychological symptom. In psychoanalysis it has been proposed that the ego calibrates a compromise between the lifting of repression and release of an impulse that then symbolically satisfies a particular wish. In contrast, paranosic gain refers to primary gain as in the development of a symptom. See Gain, primary; Gain, secondary.

ERECTILE DISORDER See Male erectile disorder.

ERIKSON, ERIK H. (1902–1994). A European-born American psychologist / psychoanalyst primarily known for his eight life stages of man. Erikson is considered a Freudian ego psychologist whose approach included a focus on socioculture. The eight stages of life are

1. *The oral sensory stage*—first year to a year and a half; task is to develop trust, while not nullifying the capacity for mistrust. This is an oblique reference to the importance of the development of reality testing.
2. *The anal-muscular stage*—eighteen months to three or four years; task is to achieve autonomy and minimize shame.
3. *The genital-locomotor stage*—three or four years of age to five or six; task is to learn initiative in the absence of guilt.
4. *The latency* stage—six to twelve years of age; task is to develop the capacity to be productive, minus feelings of inferiority. An oblique reference to the nullifying of self-doubt.
5. *The adolescence* stage—puberty to twenty; task is to achieve ego identity without any role confusion.
6. *The young adulthood stage*—twenty to thirty; task is to be open to intimacy and not to remain isolated; a reference to the ability to have a committed relationship.

7. *The middle adulthood stage*—raising children; task is to balance generativity and stagnation—in other words, how to stay productive.
8. *The late adulthood stage*—about sixty; task is to develop ego integrity minus despair—in other words, to be strong during the final stage of life.

ERIKSON, MILTON (1901–1980). Influential American psychiatrist / hypnotherapist who pioneered the use of hypnosis in psychotherapy along with developing techniques in the use of metaphor. See Hypnoanalysis.

EROS The instinct related to love or life.

EROTIC Referring to sexual excitement or libidinal interest.

EROTOGENIC MASOCHISM See Masochism.

ESP (EXTRASENSORY PERCEPTION) Never proven notion of the ability to see what others are thinking or to predict events. Synonymous with mental telepathy—the reading of other people's thoughts.

ETIOLOGY Referring to the cause of any disorder or the study of such causes.

EUPHORIA Referring to the state of well-being or happiness. In psychoanalytic usage, euphoria is usually considered when investigating sudden flights into health and / or seen as a factor in manic and otherwise elevated mood states.

EVOLUTIONARY PSYCHOPATHOLOGY Darwinian-based view of psychopathology that considers cognition and behavior in terms of adaptation to the environment.

EXCESSIVE DAYTIME SLEEPINESS (EDS) Unusual need to sleep during the day. Usually due to nighttime difficulty in sleeping or to a narcoleptic condition that disrupts normal sleep cycles. See Sleep disorders.

EXHIBITIONISM A compulsive exposing of oneself sexually to others. Considered a sexual disorder and described as a paraphilia. In derivative nonsexual form, egocentric displays within social contexts reflect the derivative nonsexual form of exhibitionism. See Paraphilia.

EXISTENTIAL PSYCHOLOGY See Phenomenology.

EXOGENOUS Disorders that are thought to be caused by anything outside the body. See Endogenous.

EXPLOSIVE DISORDER Referred to as IED or intermittent explosive disorder. This is a categorization that denotes a pattern of temper or explosive eruptions that appear intermittently and inconsistently. See Intermittent explosive disorder.

EXTERNAL OBJECT A person recognized as being different from the self or external to the self.

EXTERNALIZATION Generally equivalent to projection or to endowing others with qualities that are anathema to the self. Distinguishes self from environment.

EXTRAPUNITIVE See Punitive structure.

EXTRAVERSION OR EXTRAVERTED TYPE A Jungian formulation referring to the trait of gregariousness or social outwardness. Contrasts with introverted type. See Jung, Carl Gustav.

EYE MOVEMENT DESENSITIZATION REPROCESSING (EMDR) This relatively new treatment is an information-processing therapy especially targeted to patients with posttraumatic stress, phobias, depression, and addictions. While following the therapist's finger, the patient focuses on an image or thought or emotion. With swift eye movements, memory presumably becomes more malleable, thereby permitting positive memories to prevail over negative ones. This treatment has not yet been firmly established, although clinical anecdotal reportage has been largely positive. The theoretical assumption is that stimulated rapid eye movement can reprocess or alleviate traumatic effects of experience.

EYE-ROLL SIGN In hypnosis, the ability of the subject to be hypnotized can be determined by instruction to the subject to look upward and simultaneously lower eyelids. The extent of white showing under the cornea is said to indicate whether the subject can be easily hypnotized or not. Hysterical suggestive types, ostensibly with a great deal of white showing beneath the cornea (sanpaku), are more easily hypnotized while the opposite is said to be the case for obsessive types.

EYSENCK, HANS JURGEN (1916–1977). British psychologist who developed one of the early personality typologies and formulated the Eysenck Personality Inventory. This measurement index revealed two basic personality dimensions:

extraversion—tendency to be social;
neuroticism—tendency to experience or favor negative emotions;

A third, later-added dimension was described as

psychoticism—poor reality testing.

Eysenck favored behavioral therapy over psychodynamic approaches.

F

FABULATION A variation of the term *confabulation,* meaning confusions of meaning and expression so that solid logic is undermined. Usually fantasy material becomes inserted in memory lapses or memory distortions.

FACTITIOUS DISORDERS Feigning illness. So-called symptoms that are actually controlled by the patient fall into this category. Munchausen syndrome or hospital addictions are included here, as are all sorts of psychophysiological complaints.

FAILURE TO THRIVE Also referred to as an attachment disorder of childhood. Usually the infant is undernourished and the underdevelopment is attributed to variations of mother-infant disturbed interaction. In many such cases, anger is the emotion most implicated both in the mother's reaction to the infant as well as the infant's toward the mother, which is likely caused by the mother's resistance to any sign of autonomous response in the infant.

FAIRBAIRN, W. R. D. (1889–1964). British object relations theorist who, in contrast to a Freudian approach, postulated an ego that exists at birth. During the paranoid/schizoid period this ego fractures or splits into what Freud would consider the essential intrapsychic structure:

Central ego—equivalent to Freud's ego.
Libidinal ego—somewhat equivalent to Freud's id, but more hungry for the object rather than for instinctual release.
Antilibidinal ego—somewhat equivalent to Freud's superego, but the anitilibidinal ego attacks the libidinal ego's need for the object. It is always impulsive, reactive, and retaliatory.

Fairbairn minimized instinct. Rather, the relationship between the self and the object was now seen as a function of experience by the self with the object. Thus, ego became for Fairbairn the source of its own energy. Problems for the infant with respect to faulty subject-object connection would cause later depressive reactions. Fairbairn also pointed out the the abuser's psychology as a derivative and repetition of personal childhood abuse.

FALSE SELF See Winnicott, D. W.

FALSIFICATION, RETROSPECTIVE Insertion and elaboration of detail into memories, so that the remembered event can have a meaning corresponding to the current need of the subject, in contrast to faithfully reflecting the original event. Seen in paranoid schizophrenic patients who utilize such falsification in the service of the delusional aim. This is also a factor that must be examined in the retrieval of memory with respect to the claim of incestuous or other historical sexual abuse.

FAMILY ROMANCE The child's sense that his parents are not really his parents. Rather, the child feels adopted, and that the original parents were of a higher or greater station.

FAMILY THERAPY The psychotherapeutic treatment of the entire family system. One of the goals in such treatment is to shed light on the contrast between the apparently problematic person in the family against the actual one (who may not be apparent). Thus the ostensible patient and the actual patient may not be the same person. In a family therapy systems, the therapeutic strategy is to penetrate the entrenched pathological pattern of the family by reordering patterns of communication. There are many approaches to family treatment including the use of systems theory, communication theory, structural family therapy, solution-focused therapy, and others. Contributors to the metapsychology as well as treatment approaches in family therapy include Ackerman, Bateson, Bowen, Framo, A. M. Freedman, Haley, Jackson, A.I. Kaplan, Minuchin, Rabkin, B. Saddock, V. Saddock, Sager, Satir, Singer, Spitz, Watzlawick, Whitaker.

FANTASY A product of imagining some scenario, usually in which the subject gratifies a wish. Compensatory needs are frequently the subject of such scenarios. The more one is withdrawn, the more time is devoted to fantasy life, so to speak, behind the line. See Line, The.

FEAR Considered by most personality theorists to be a primary emotion connoting a flight impulse. Thus, it may be said that fear wants to flee. Personality theorists have also found that fear-mixed traits are considered to be socially desirable, in contrast, for example, to anger-mixed traits, which are considered to be socially undesirable. Caution (a fear-mixed trait) is an example of the former, while argumentativeness (an anger-mixed trait) is an example of the latter. Clinically, in extreme cases, fear is seen as a component of dread or phobia. In psychoanalysis fear is implicated in guilt or in superego issues of conscience.

FEEBLEMINDEDNESS Underdevelopment of mental capacity. Deficient or even retarded cognitive functioning.

FEEDING PROBLEM This is not a reference to an anorectic diagnosis, although the child becomes quite finicky about food and eating.

FEELING More or less synonymous with emotion, affect, mood, and empathy. See Emotion.

FEELING TYPE See Jung, Carl Gustav.

FELDENKRAIS, MOSHE (1904–1984). Ukrainian-born Israeli engineer. See Body-focused therapy.

FELLATIO Oral sex performed on a male.

FEMININE MASOCHISM See Masochism.

FENICHEL, OTTO (1897–1946). Viennese psychoanalyst best known for his popular psychoanalytic text, *The Psycho-*

analytic Theory of Neurosis. Considered psychoanalysis the core of a hypothesized reformulation of psychodynamic psychology—as a dialectical materialistic psychology derived from his Marxist orientation.

FERENCZI, SANDOR (1873–1933). Hungarian psychoanalyst who formulated what is known as active therapy. The orientation called active therapy was also used by Stekel in his work, and by Rosen as well. Briefly analyzed by Freud but created own set of therapeutic postulates that Freud found anathema to the enterprise of psychoanalysis. Ferenczi promoted active contact with patients that included a more reciprocal flow of communication. He anticipated the human potential movement; his focus on a caring attitude led him to provide patients with love, of which they were presumably deprived in childhood. At one point he even tried, but later abandoned, what he called mutual analysis (analyst and patient take turns with each role), in order to counteract the hierarchical, vertical, and thus ostensibly undemocratic nature of the analyst-patient relationship. Ferenczi analyzed and influenced Melanie Klein, Michael Balint, and Clara Thompson. Contributors to reviews and analyses of Ferenczi's work include Aron, Brabant, Dupont, Gedo, Harris, Haynal, Loland, Rachman, and Thompson. The following is a sample of Ferenczi's formulations.

Blocking acting out—designed to increase fantasy flow.

Confusion of tongues—communication between parent and child in which the child is confronted with seduction from the parent rather than tenderness, which is what the child actually craves.

Empathy—called the rule of empathy, designed to focus on reflection of, and congruence with, the patient's feelings.

Forced fantasies—this concept was formulated in response to his experience with patients who reported few or no fantasies. He found that this paucity of fantasy was a result of an absence of sufficient affect; therefore Ferenczi devised methods to generate fantasy in these patients, the purpose of which was to cultivate the personality in order to enrich the panoply of affect. This was also a method to liberate negative feelings; a formal process of intervention where the therapist issues prohibitions in the session designed to undermine resistance.

Regression—the attempt to use regression in service of the therapy—akin to regression in service of the ego.

Relaxation therapy—an attempt to create a more healing ambience.

Role playing—designed to generate more opportunity for the patient to work on conflict.

Treatment of phobias—use of confrontation techniques to treat phobias.

FESTINGER, LEON (1919–1989). American social psychologist. Although not specifically functioning as a clinician, nevertheless, Festinger's formulation of cognitive dissonance contains important implications for understanding behavior—that there is inconsistency in the beliefs people hold so that they change their beliefs to correspond to and fit their behavior rather than the other way around. This insight has been helpful to cognitive behavioral theorists and therapists as well as to psychoanalysts and the broad spectrum of relational therapists. See Cognitive dissonance theory.

FETISH A focus on some symbol that connotes a magical and compelling interest for the subject, usually inspired by, connected to, and directed toward an obsessive love object and infused with sexual significance.

FIELD DEPENDENT Reliance on outside forces to define the self.

FIGHT-FLIGHT GROUP See Assumption group.

FIVE FACTOR MODEL Also known as the Big Five Factors (of personality). Shown statistically to apply to a wide array of clinical situations. In interpersonal theory, an approach to the study and understanding of the organization of personality traits. The model is utilized to show that people vary to one extent or another in each of these factors: *openness, conscientiousness, extraversion, agreeableness, and neuroticism (OCEAN).*

1. *openness to experience*—appreciation for art, invention, imagination;

2. *conscientiousness*—ability to plan, to have self-discipline, to achieve;
3. *extraversion*—being social, enjoying positive emotions;
4. *agreeableness*—showing cooperation and empathy rather than antagonism;
5. *neuroticism*—given to experiencing negative emotions like anger, anxiety, and depression.

Contributors to the study of this model include Costa, Digman, Goldberg, McCrae, and Saucier.

FIXATION A psychoanalytic term denoting a prevalent focus infused with libidinous impulse and formed into obsessive preoccupation and compulsive activity. The object of the fixation is the one toward whom the subject is cathected; that is, the one who is invested with an entrenched transferential energy. The presence of a fixation implies some degree of arrested development insofar as a fixation keeps a person fixed at one point regardless of the march of time. See Cathexis.

FLAGELLATION Physical punishment toward self or another in the form of whipping. Clinically, voluntary flagellation is understood as an act that satisfies a sadomasochistic sexual intent.

FLASHBACK A condition seen in posttraumatic stress disorder patients, often among war veterans and disaster survivors experiencing a mental sensation of a sudden recurrence of the traumatic experience. See Posttraumatic stress disorder.

FLAT AFFECT Emotional tone or intonation that lacks any inflection. Seen in schizophrenic individuals and one of the four *A*s developed by Bleuler to diagnose schizophrenia. Flat affect is noticed because responses to mild or severe circumstances seem not to be differentiated in the person's affective tone. In historical psychiatric diagnostic nomenclature was pathognomonic of simple schizophrenia. See Bleuler, Eugen; Schizophrenia.

FLIGHT INTO HEALTH Usually occurring as a result of the relationship of patient to therapist. The patient has not actually recovered as a result of a resolution of conflict. Rather, a compensatory transferential improvement of symptoms seems to qualify as a recovery of emotional health because of the sudden (flight) disappearance of pathology based on the positive therapeutic encounter.

FLIGHT INTO ILLNESS See Disease, flight into.

FLIGHT OF IDEAS Usually, but not always a manifestation of internal manic pressure within manic-depressive psychosis, manic phase. Such a person can talk continuously, going from idea to idea without any real development of any one of them. The intent of the person exhibiting such flight of ideas is not at all derived from an interest in the give and take of any relationship. Instead this symptom arises out of a psychopathological interior pressure insofar as such a person needs to generate continuous external stimulation. With respect to differential diagnosis, the need to generate external stimulation in the manic personality is not manipulative the way it is in the psychopathic personality; in addition, minor examples of such flights of ideas can also be seen in anxious individuals who are not psychotic but experience exaggerated social tensions. Thus the flight of ideas in the socially tense person can take the counterphobic form of talking a lot. Otherwise, the flight of ideas is also seen in individuals with schizophrenic disorders.

FLOODING Technique used in behavior therapy and cognitive behavior therapy to reduce catastrophic fears (extreme anxiety, phobias, PTSD) and, by imagining in vivid detail the feared scene and accompanying irrational thoughts, followed where possible by *in vivo practice* (real-life exposure).

Cognitive flooding—a type of paradoxical technique that involves having clients repeatedly state aloud their irrational thoughts until satiated (bored, tired, annoyed) in order to decrease their frequency and intensity. See Systematic desensitization.

FOLIE À DEUX A phrase meaning that two people share a common pathology. Also known as double insanity. Diagnostically, has been used to describe general psychotic behavior and paranoid delusional thinking whereby one person's influence is effective in influencing the other, assuming the same kind of thinking in the other, or, so to speak, buying into it. Since suggestibility is implicated in the transmission of the pathology, a latent component of the pathology contains at least some hysteric elements. On the manifest level the characterological fabric of the personality, rather than appearing suggestible, seems rather rigid.

FONAGY, PETER (1952–). British psychologist / psychoanalyst. As a researcher and child analyst investigated the psychology of psychic reality, borderline psychopathology, the psychology of attachment, the operation of affect regulation, and data on mental / cognitive development from birth.

FORCED FANTASIES See Ferenczi, Sandor.

FORENSIC PSYCHOLOGY A reference to the legal dimension in the practice of psychological health services. Practically speaking, usually involves expert court testimony by a psychiatrist, psychologist, or other mental health expert.

FORWARD EDGE TRANSFERENCE See Transference.

FREE ASSOCIATION Freud's assumption that ideas brought forth in the absence of concentration, with willingness on the part of the patient to report these ideas freely, will lead to the emergence of important unconscious material (conflict) and will also tend to minimize therapeutic resistance. Provides one rationale for use of the couch in psychoanalytic treatment insofar as it is thought that the patient will be less self-monitoring when not experiencing the stimulus of the therapist face to face.

FREE-FLOATING ANXIETY See Anxiety, free-floating.

FREUD, ANNA (1895–1982). Daughter of Sigmund Freud. Austrian-born British psychoanalyst, considered the founder of child psychoanalysis. She is best known for her work in child therapy as well as for her focus on the organization of defense mechanisms. Her ideas on the ego in its relation to id and superego influenced further investigation into the function and infrastructure of the ego with environmental stimuli. She also supported the theoretical position of drive theory as the seminal variable in motivation and believed that earliest satisfactions comprised the basis of future object relations.

FREUD, SIGMUND (1856–1939). The founder of psychoanalysis. Born in Austria. Proposed and developed concepts of the unconscious, resistance, defenses generally and repression specifically, transference, as well as an entire lexicon of concatenated concepts, all interstitially related in a prismlike effect, emitting a profound variety of insights into the human psyche as well as into the infrastructural psyche of society. In his magnum opus—*The Interpretation of Dreams*—published in 1900 (eight editions were published up to 1930), in the preface to the third revised English edition (1932), he stated about his own discoveries that "insight such as this falls to one's lot but once in a lifetime." His notion that acting out is an attempt to do something rather than to know something is the cornerstone of psychoanalysis itself. This concept distinguishes psychiatry from psychoanalysis insofar as, from a psychiatric vantage point, the definition of acting out would emphasize any pathological "doing" or delinquent behavior, whereas, in psychoanalytic understanding, acting out reveals a dynamic that includes defenses, resistance, repression, and an entire host of collateral psychodynamic concepts. It is said that the three blows to man's egotism were dealt by Copernicus, Darwin, and Freud. In discovering that the sun doesn't revolve around the earth, Copernicus struck the first blow. Darwin later asserted that we evolved from lower forms of life and that our closest relatives are apes. In both cases, we realized we were not as special as we thought we were. The final and perhaps fatal blow to man's ego came from Freud, who told us that we didn't know our own minds (meaning to many, no doubt, that we were not nearly as smart as we thought we were). Although there have been many variations on the Freudian psychoanalytic sensibility, none have been fashioned into as powerful a theory as his psychoanalytic smorgasbord itself; in considering the scientific criterion for what makes the most powerful theory, scientists agree that the theory that accounts for the widest array of phenomena with reference to the fewest number of variables will be the most powerful theory—in this sense psychoanalysis triumphs. It should be noted, however, that in the past thirty years there has been an outpouring of work, concepts, theory, and research in the domains of self psychology and the relational therapies as well as in cognitive behavior therapy, with treatment successes purporting to validate a great deal of the work. It is cognitive behavior therapy that is now the alternative to psychodynamic and psychoanalytic treatment—or perhaps visa versa. Be that as it may, and notwithstanding proclamations to the contrary, psychoanalysis is very much alive. Cognitive behavior psychology is now the dominant force in psychology departments nationwide, although psychoanalysis is the lens of choice in literature departments, anthropology departments, and other social science and humanities programs—all because of the consensus that psychoanalysis is the template of insight that plumbs the depths of the human psyche and experience and makes available the same template for understanding broad social-psychological and sociological phenomena. Freud's body of work can be viewed with respect to a few subtheories that unify his conception of psychopathology. Greenspan's summary of these are

adaptive theory—relation of ego to environment with respect to reality testing and secondary process;
economic theory—drive energy striving for expression and accessibility to consciousness with respect to behavior;
genetic theory—history correlated to current behavior;
psychosexual theory—relation of character formation to stages of development;
structural theory—system of intrapsychic forces—ego / id / superego;
topographical theory—unconscious, preconscious, conscious.

Freud also developed a character typology based on psychosexual developmental stages:

Oral stage—consists of both oral passive (passive-dependent character style) and oral aggressive (character traits of cruelty and hostility).
Anal stage—consists of both anal expulsive (character traits of messiness and disorderliness) and anal retentive

(character traits of orderliness, stinginess, withholding of emotional warmth).

Phallic stage—consists of phallic exhibitionistic impulses (ambition, exhibitionism, narcissism, and pride, along with sensitivity to deflation and lack of appreciation from others). Castration anxiety is the central concern of this stage, with self-esteem always in focus. Passive-aggressive patterns obtain.

Oedipal stage—with the oedipal conflict, the family triangle is the central issue; that is, with closeness to the opposite gender parent and hostility to the same gender parent. Traits include loyalty to the oedipal object (decreasing the probability for mature relating), competitiveness, and the need for conquest.

Freudian psychoanalysis was the dominant dynamic psychology of most of the twentieth century, supported by countless numbers of theoreticians, authors, researchers, teachers, and practitioners. Scores of individuals can be represented by the following sample, along with a host of others who may be found as separate entries herein. Among these contributors are Arlow, Brenner, Eitingon, Federn, Fenichel, Jones, Kriss, Reich, Reik, Sachs, Stekel, Waelder. James Strachey is the editor of *The Standard Edition of the Complete Psychological Works of Sigmund Freud.*

In the latter part of the twentieth century and on into the twenty-first, theories and treatment technologies have evolved out of newer conceptualizations with respect to the more relational schools of thought, which are focused differently than Freudian drive theory. Yet they stand on the shoulders of the psychoanalysis of repression, the unconscious, transference, and overall psychodynamic understanding. These newer approaches have been inviting greater and greater interest and have already gained ascendancy among many younger and some older thinkers and practitioners. These are the relational theorists, among whom are counted object relationists, intersubjectivists, and some hybrids such as the psychoanalytic ego psychologists. Such individuals include Aron, Bacal, Balint,

Beebe, Bion, Buirski, Ehrenberg, Fairbairn, Fosshage, Grotstein, Guntrip, Harris, Hartmann, Horner, Jacobson, Kavaler-Adler, Kernberg, Klein, Kohut, Lacan, Lachmann, Mahler, Masterson, Mitchell, Ogden, Seinfeld, Stolorow, Strupp, Winnicott.

FREUDIAN SLIP A misstep in speech that reveals underlying true feelings, motives, or thinking. See Parapraxis.

FREUD'S SYNDROME Freud's stunning focus on the phenomenon of repression and its unfolding invited the coining of the phrase "Freud's syndrome." This means that a so-called repressive irresistibility exists, where incredible symptoms such as projections of the most skewed fantasies and impulses imply that the cause of such derivative and manifest material has as its source-motive that which is housed in the unconscious. Of course, this "housed" material in the unconscious is protected, first and foremost, by repression and, second, by resistance. The job of the resistance is to support repression. Thus, with respect to repression, Freud's syndrome is essential to the understanding of pathology and all symptom formation. Freud's syndrome essentially represents the life of the unconscious.

FRIGIDITY, SEXUAL A woman's difficulty in achieving orgasm, although not necessarily never achieving orgasm. In frigidity there can be varying degrees of difficulty. The corresponding difficulty in men is termed impotence.

FROMM, ERICH (1900–1980). European-born American psychologist. Developed a typology of neurotic styles that individuals use to manage alienation. Thus it is implied that people seek safety and security. Seeking community with others offers such security provided that integrity is not compromised. This community with others develops altruism. Fromm postulated five personality or orientation types. These are divided into four that are nonproductive and one that is productive. The nonproductive types include

the receptive orientation—security is sought passively from others;

the exploitative orientation—security is sought forcefully from others;

the hoarding orientation—security is sought by saving whatever one possesses;

the marketing orientation—security is sought through salesmanship.

The one productive type is

the productive orientation—security is gained through effort and self-actualization.

Fromm may be considered an anthropological psychoanalyst, somewhat similar to Abraham Kardiner. In Fromm's case however, his gaze is on an existential community phenomenon in which healthy functioning very much depends on the success of one's cultural embeddedness. Love, for example, is not considered an emotion so much as it derives from an interpersonal capacity and includes facets of caring, responsibility, respect, and knowledge. Similarly, guilt and shame result from a disunited human existence; that is to say, separated from the society and culture. Fromm was one of the founders, in 1946, of the William Alanson White Institute, a psychoanalytic institute influenced by the philosophy of Sandor Ferenczi. Other founders include Clara Thompson (famed interpersonal psychoanalyst), Harry Stack Sullivan (credited with developing the interpersonal school), and Frieda Fromm-Reichmann (who focused on treatment with schizophrenic patients).

FROMM-REICHMANN, FRIEDA (1890–1957). European-born American psychoanalyst well known for her work in schizophrenia, especially with reference to her positive, hopeful insistence that schizophrenic individuals could be treated in psychotherapy. Early in her career she worked with Kurt Goldstein treating brain-injured patients. She also worked with Erich Fromm (whom she married), and was deeply influenced by Freud as well as Harry Stack Sullivan. She was one of the founders of the William Alanson White Psychoanalytic Institute. Fromm-Reichmann considered herself to be an interpersonalist / psychoanalyst who, even with schizophrenic patients, was optimistic with respect to eventually being able to establish a more normal transference relationship and thereby repair various facets of the patient's disturbance.

FRONTAL EXECUTIVE CONTROL OF MESOCORTICAL AND MESOLIMBIC "SEEKING" SYSTEMS According to Kaplan-Solms and Solms, in neuropsychoanalysis, the loss of such systems produces primary process thinking as exemplified in dreams and confabulations.

FRONTAL LOBE EXECUTIVE CONTROL SYSTEMS According to Solms and Turnbull, and in the domain of neuropsychoanalysis, this is the biological source of secondary process or reality-oriented thinking. Further, this usually applies to nonlimbic left dorsolateral (as opposed to right orbitofrontal) activity. Primary process cognition is the product of right brain operations; not just a release of left brain secondary process cognition. In other words, there are two frontal systems, not one.

FROZEN WATCHFULNESS A kind of vigilance seen in children who have experienced abuse. The frozen watchfulness is a physical appearance whereby the child scans and fixes its gaze on particular elements of any circumstance and conveys a sense of guardedness.

FRUSTRATION In a clinical sense, always related to an abridged wish and usually hyphenated with aggression. That is, that when frustrated, a wish will have been adumbrated and the resulting sense of disempowerment will have created anger. The axiom is that helplessness (or disempowerment) always breeds rage. Thus, frustration will produce a sudden sense of disempowerment and then generate anger in response to this disempowerment, which in turn will create just as sudden a sense of the possibility of reempowerment. This is so because anger is an expostulation of power—frequently an empowerment. The frustration-aggression hypothesis is at the center of this dynamic. In child development, maturation as an ongoing process very much depends on the child's ability to tolerate frustration and correspondingly to focus on more long-range goals rather than always feeling persuaded by the needs of the moment. In cases where there is significant developmental arrest, the child frequently responds episodically to each and every circumstance rather than being able to postpone immediate needs for gratification. See Symptom.

FRUSTRATION-AGGRESSION HYPOTHESIS Frustration always leads to aggressive feelings and, depending how the subject manages anger, may either lead to the expostulation of the aggression or to its repression.

FRUSTRATION TOLERANCE A measure of ego strength. Relates to the ability to tolerate thwarted goals. The better one tolerates frustration, the better one's ego strength. Psychoanalytically relates to the ascendancy of the ego over the instincts.

FUGUE A clinical condition in which the subject can dissociate current whereabouts and drift to other geographical areas or simply become distracted by a variety of random stimuli, unaware, all the while, of the normal continuity and / or identity of one's life. See Psychogenic fugue.

FUNCTION ENGRAM See Jung, Carl Gustav.

FUNCTIONAL NEGATIVE FEELINGS See Dysfunctional negative feelings.

G

GAIN, PRIMARY Freedom from anxiety is the primary gain of a symptom. Also referred to as paranosic gain.

GAIN, SECONDARY Individuals gain special attention from illness or other disabling circumstances, and such focus on the subject by others is experienced as gratifying. Referred to also as epinosic gain. Correlates to conditions of dependency on parental or authority figures.

GAIT, STUTTERING An awkward hesitating gait attributed to hysterical reactions. Observed in psychotic patients. Similar to stuttering in speech.

GALEN, CLAUDIUS (AD 129–199). Ancient Greek physician who underscored biological approaches to assessing personality. Predicted that manifestations of psychopathology correlated to brain damage and influenced the idea of a neurological basis of behavior.

GANSER SYNDROME Also referred to as the nonsense syndrome, meaning that the patient offers tangential responses, or incomplete ones, or those that are slightly off target, the purpose of which is to curry favor with authority by appearing to be an innocent. The differential diagnosis is usually one of hysterical versus malingering (psychopathic): is it that the person is truly, albeit unconsciously, creating such confusion, or is it that the person is consciously manipulative?

GELINEAU'S SYNDROME Referring to narcolepsy. Named for a French neurologist, J. B. E. Gelineau (1859–1906). See Narcolepsy.

GENDER IDENTITY Refers generally to the extent to which a person is certain of his or her particular gender (feels secure in that gender), both with regard to role as well as to physical attributes.

GENDER IDENTITY DISORDER A persistent cross-gender identification.

GENEALOGY Referring to ancestral lineage.

GENERAL ADAPTATION SYNDROME (GAS) Postulated by Hans Selye (Austrian-Hungarian physician (1902–1987) as a way to understand the phenomenon and vicissitudes of stress and to reduce stress and tension. Selye's focus on stress consists of three phases: the alarm reaction, resistance, and exhaustion. This means that the person defends against stress in a pivotal crisis through the use of an adaptative effort, which he identified as the general adaptation syndrome—comprising the following processes:

Alarm reaction stage—the immediate reaction to the stressor generating fight / flight reactions, a reaction characterized by an emotional and physiological shock to the system along with countercompensatory responses.

Resistance stage—an adaptation stage in which the body attempts to stabilize itself, using extra energy to adapt to the stress and thereby taxing the body's energy reserves, even affecting the immune system.

Exhaustion—prolonged adaptation to stress can exhaust one's resources; the appearance of symptoms based upon a breakdown of the body's resistance—including sleeplessness, loss of appetite, irritability, and general fatigue. See Selye, Hans; Stress.

GENERAL SYSTEMS THEORY The idea that the structure of any system reveals its operation. Such structure includes how the system utilizes its mechanisms to calibrate interactions and, specifically with respect to psychopathology, the balance of impulses versus controls. Therefore it is the study of complex systems with respect to the internal consistency of the theoretical network, also referred to as the nomological network. Systems theory has been utilized in group and family therapy theory and is influenced by the work of scientists from a wide spectrum of disciplines. Contributors include Bateson, Bertalanffy, Mead, and Prigogine.

GENETIC In biology, referring to transfer of characteristics—parent to child: the study of heredity. In psychoanalytic discourse, usually refers to psychological-emotional development.

GENITAL CHARACTER In psychoanalytic thinking, this is a person who has reached mature adjustment by resolving conflict at earlier stages of psychosexual development—oral, anal, phallic, and oedipal.

GENITAL STAGE Refers to the psychoanalytic concept of mature development at the adult stage. See Genital character.

GENOGRAM Showing the genealogy of the family tree.

GENOTYPE Referring to individual predisposition of characteristics, despite environmental conditions.

GENUINENESS See Rogers, Carl.

GERIATRICS Referring to disorders of the elderly.

GESTALT PSYCHOLOGY A conception of the whole as being greater than its parts (actually the whole is different than its parts). Gestalt psychology, influenced by Max Wertheimer, posits a brain that is holistic. This view revealed principles of perception, as, for example, in the way objects are perceived. Principles of gestalt systems include

1. *emergence*—tendency to see the whole rather than its parts;
2. *invariance*—objects are recognized despite any possible spatial rotation;

3. *multistability*—if there are alternative percepts available, the subject will shift back and forth between them;
4. *reification*—a generative aspect of perception by which the subject, through spatial organizing, makes more out of actual stimuli.

GESTALT THERAPY An experiential system of theory and psychotherapy treatment emphasizing the person as a whole organism in contrast to seeing the person as a part object. The theory also emphasizes that the individual will want to complete any incomplete picture in order to see the whole percept. Concretely, Gestalt therapy is an expressive form of therapy in which the patient may act out (in the denotative sense of performing) particular roles and then consider feelings regarding these roles in the here and now. Utilizes expressive techniques from a host of psychotherapy modalities. Promoted by Fritz Perls. See Perls, Fritz.

GILL, MERTON M. (1914–1994). American psychiatrist who was influential in the twentieth-century distillation of psychoanalytic principles and the definition of psychoanalysis itself. These principles also referred to diagnostic formulations. The group of psychologists engaged in this dialogue included Holt, G. Klein, Rappaport, Schafer, and Wallerstein.

GILLES DE LA TOURETTE SYNDROME Named for Georges Gilles de la Tourette, European physician (1857–1904). Usually referred to simply as Tourette syndrome. Characterized by a variety of tics (facial, body, voice). The symptoms begin in childhood and can appear up to mid adolescence and beyond. Has gained notoriety mostly because, in some cases, the tic is expressed through the use of extravagant and inappropriate profanity. It is an inherited neurological disorder, at times associated with attention deficit disorder and influenced epigenetically by environmental stimuli. It is part of a category labeled *Tic Disorders* as listed in the *DSM* nosology of the American Psychiatric Association.

GLOBAL ASSESSMENT OF FUNCTIONING (GAF SCALE) *DSM* classification of the extent of maladjustment.

GLOBAL DETERIORATION SCALE (GDS) An assessment of cognitive deterioration in elderly patients based upon performance behavior. Results can point to both minor and major changes in mental status.

GLOBUS HYSTERICUS The sensation of choking, which feels like a globe blocking the passageway in the throat. Seen as a hysterical symptom attributed to sexual ambivalence involving an attraction / rejection conflict. Theoretically, the choking symptom is said to reflect underlying anger regarding some unrealized wish (perhaps regarding unrequited love) and a corresponding sense of disempowerment (because of the thwarted wish) that then generates the anger, which in turn is then repressed. The sensation of blockage in the throat is now an imagined somatized symptom that represents the blockage of the relationship (unrequited). See Symptom.

GLOSSOLALIA The creation of phrases or sentences comprised of nonsense syllables constituting the creation of new yet nonmeaning neologisms. Designed to simulate actual language. Sometimes seen in schizophrenia as word salads, which reflect severe disturbance.

GOOD ENOUGH MOTHER See Winnicott, D. W.

GOOD OBJECT Can be found discussed by Freud and Rado, but extensively developed by Klein and Fairbairn. The object relations notion here refers to an object (person) who is internalized as a strength object supporting ego functioning and, thereby, from a psychoanalytic perspective, also delimiting the effects of the hypothesized death instinct. The good object protects the subject from threats both from without and from within. It refers to a facet of Klein's stages of mental development and is associated with what Klein refers to as the paranoid-schizoid position, in which the infant is presumably defended against its own death instinct—and whereby its own aggression is projected to an object (person), while the breast is internalized as a good object.

GOODENOUGH TEST Florence Goodenough, American psychologist (1886–1959), developed a method to measure the intelligence of children through an analysis of the child's drawing of a human figure. This measurement can also be utilized in conjunction with the Machover figure drawing test developed by Karen Machover to assess personality. See Machover Draw a Person Test (DAP).

GRANDIOSITY Usually associated with paranoia insofar as the person becomes megalomaniacal, attributing major powers of influence to the self. Magnified self-importance. In paranoid schizophrenia the grandiosity is labeled a delusion of grandeur. Its fraternal twin delusion is labeled a delusion of persecution. Also present in pathological narcissism. See Delusion.

GRAPHOLOGY The analysis of cursive writing (handwriting) as a way of assessing personality and understanding diagnostic organization of the personality.

GRAZIANO, ROBERTA (1941–) Author of studies on clinical work with survivors of trauma. Professor and director, Aging and Health Program, and former associate dean, Hunter College School of Social Work, City University of New York, member, editorial board, *Dictionary of Psychopathology.*

GROUP THERAPY Several individuals coming together in a group for a psychotherapeutic purpose. In clinical settings, psychodynamic groups will typically consist of six to eight or nine members plus the therapist. The group meets on a once-per-week basis and is usually allotted ninety minutes. In a psychoanalytic group the membership interacts on a first-name basis so that anonymity is reasonably assured. Members are encouraged to engage with one another in a verbal interactive frame, in the here and now of the group, and are discouraged from too much reportage of actual events of their lives outside the group. The here and now interactions also enable interpretive opportunities that can resonate for each group member with respect to personal history—the there and then. Individuals are also discouraged from any outside contact among or between members, the purpose of which is to retain the group's tension within it and not permit this tension to dissipate through other member-to-member personal contact. This discouragement of outside contact also discourages subgrouping or the forming of tacit alliances between members within the group, which would necessarily contribute to an aggregate of resistance to the therapeutic work of the group. The therapist will try to identify group themes, that is, themes that seem to organize what the overall interactions mean. In addition, the therapist interprets transference of individual members of the group. In this sense, historical material of members is also introduced. Further, although the basic model underlying the work of each member of the group has been thought to reflect original nuclear family issues of these members, it is becoming clear, according to Kellerman, that the true basic model of the group is the primary relationship of each member: how one functions in the group is an exact replica (isomorphic) of how that person actually behaves in the primary relationship—or how that person would be in any future primary relationship, marriage, or partnership. Thus, through the work in the group, the group members can begin to palpably experience themselves as though in primary relationships and correspondingly see how they actually feel in a relationship and where they might be able to change or improve their interaction with a partner. A good amount of work in a group could occupy a period of about three years, although individuals can do ongoing work for much longer periods. Other groups such as Gestalt groups, psychodrama groups, or short-term goal-oriented groups have ground rules that are quite different from those of the psychodynamically oriented clinical group described here. Theoretically, the group experience is a more direct confrontation with one's characterological organization (one's entrenched personality trait configuration), in contrast to individual psychodynamic psychotherapy, which is thought to address anxiety issues and the variety of stresses people experience that bring them into therapy in the first place, and connect these to historical relationships of the person's childhood. Contributors to group therapy theory and practice have included Agazarian, Alonso, Aronson, Bales, Bion, Block-Lewis, Durkin, Fieldsteel, Foulkes, Frankel, Freud, Ganzarain, Glatzer, Grotjahn, Kadis, Kauff, Kellerman, Kibel, LeBon, Lewin, Liff, Livingston, Moreno, Nicholas, Ormont, Perls, Pines, Rachman,

Rutan, Scheidlinger, Schwartz, Spotnitz, Stone, Wong, Wright, and Yalom. Slavson and A. Wolf are credited with pioneering this modality.

GUILT Typically defined as the result of forbidden pleasures. In personality trait theory, guilt is thought to be composed of the emotions pleasure, sorrow, and fear. In psychoanalytic understanding, it contains strong superego influence standing against impulses that threaten to gain the ascendancy. Where there is guilt, anxiety usually appears on top, but it may be that what is more basic in the dynamics of guilt is a deeply repressed and etched anger toward a particular person. Where there is guilt, a sense of transgression will be present, although, again, it is suspected that anger lurks beneath. Thus, in psychoanalytic understanding, guilt is a function of the conflict between superego pressure, on the one hand, and aggressive and sexual instincts, on the other—a displacement of the conflict between parent and child. Practically speaking, reparation addresses guilt. In rational emotive behavior theory, guilt is seen as resulting from two cognitions: "I should not have done this bad thing and, as a result, I am a bad person." Clients are instead taught to "damn the deed, but not the doer," leading to regret and motivation to do better next time.

GUNTRIP, HARRY (1901–1975). British psychologist who synthesized the work of several of the object relations theorists—Klein, Winnicott, Fairbairn. Focused on schizoid experience with respect to the withdrawal of energy from the external world into the interior world of internal objects. Thus, the object became crucial for ego development—that is, Guntrip located the self at the nuclear center of all of psychoanalytic theory. For Guntrip, the ego had much in common with Kohut's self psychology. Guntrip felt that when the schizoid experience is further regressed, hopelessness and despair would follow. As a construct, such regression is crucial to Guntrip, because he proposed that it can deplete the personality. The way to resist that depletion is by attaching to objects and nourishing object relations. For Guntrip, the profound phenomenon in psychopathology is withdrawal.

H

HAIR PULLING Known as trichotillomania, and classified in the psychiatric nosology as an impulse disorder. Psychoanalytically related to exhibitionism and considered to be a masturbatory equivalent. Hair is pulled from the head and pubic area; even eyelashes can be pulled and pulled out. Psychodynamically, trichotillomania may be derived from a strong oedipal/incestuous drama (usually not acted out, although seductively close) that overwhelms the fantasy life, albeit unconsciously. The urge to pull hair becomes obsessive and then compulsively acted out. It is thought to be highly correlated to guilt regarding imagined or real infractions—usually sexual. Hypothetically, also may be a result of repressed anger and exasperation with the seductive parent or parent figure. Hence, pulling your hair out can be a result of a paroxysm of seductive provocation—getting rid of the person

HALEY, JAY (1908–2007). American psychologist. Known for his work in family therapy and in the investigations into psychotherapy process. Pioneered work in systemic family therapy. See Family therapy.

HALLOWEEN EFFECT Supposed increase in activity (hyperactivity) from the ingestion of sugar or sugar products.

HALLUCINATION The perception or experience of something outside the self where no such thing exists. This perception can involve all of the senses including, most commonly, the visual, auditory, and even olfactory. It is different from a delusion, which is most commonly defined as a false belief, or different from an illusion, which is defined as a mistaken perception caused by actual stimuli. Psychoanalytically, hallucinations are seen as wish fulfillment. Included in the variants of hallucinations are

Hallucination, blank—experiences of an oblique nature in that the person is affected by generalized rhythmiclike influences that are inanimate and, moreover, constitute seemingly mechanical phenomena. An example would be a person feeling an undulating sense of gravity waves.

Hallucination, hypnagogic—See Narcolepsy.

Hallucination, negative—usually referring to the hypnotic state in which, through suggestion, the subject does not see an object that is really present.

HAPLOLOGY Rapid speech in which words are condensed, as in the squashing of syllables. Usually seen in manic states or in severe anxiety states.

HARTMANN, HEINZ (1894–1970). European-born American psychiatrist / psychoanalyst known as one of the founders of ego psychology. Ego psychology is a personality development theory concerned with the psychology of internalizations, or identifications with so-called ego models such as nuclear family members, and corresponds to the field of object relations theory. Hartmann followed Freud's focus on instinct but gave to the ego its own instinctual energy. He also felt that the adaptation to reality was the salient criterion from which to assess psychopathology. Following are his five ego functions, which have been considered useful in the assessment of cognitive functioning and reality testing:

Primary autonomous function—impairment of this function involves the level at which distinct and gross perceptual distortions appear.

Secondary autonomous function—impairment of this function implies a pathological interference in directed thought and the possible breakthrough of primary process material.

Integrative function—impairment of this function implies that, in the face of intact reality testing, a problem in the regulation of instinctual drives and feelings and the management of anxiety is in question. It is an issue of dubious control over impulse.

Synthetic function—impairment here suggests that ambiguity with regard to goals is not easily tolerated and that therefore goal achievement is less likely.

Adaptive function—impairment here calls into question the extent to which inner resources can be empoweringly integrated for high achievement.

Hartmann proposed that all of psychopathology can be addressed through the analysis of such ego functioning. It was his way of developing an adaptational ego psychology, also positioning ego function centrally in psychoanalysis, which was essentially a broadening of Freudian theory toward being adaptational as well as biological.

HATE A compound emotion consisting of a combination of anger and disgust. In psychoanalytic thinking Freud considered hate to be derived from the death instinct. Hate is also inextricably tied to ego, insofar as assault to the ego—as in humiliation—will, in almost all instances, generate rejection behavior (disgust), and at least the wish to attack (anger). Hate is also primarily generated by scapegoating, as well as secondarily contributing to a compounding of scapegoating, inviting violence and vengeance. With respect to ego defenses, hate is connected to the defenses of projection and displacement. In this way the self is protected from feelings of self-revulsion, and the hated object, rather than being the self, becomes located in the other.

HEADACHE, CLUSTER A migraine or migrainelike headache usually characterized by eye and head pain. The pain can be sustained for long periods and continue to intermittently occur, even for twenty-four hours. The pain can then again continue for days or even weeks. Can periodically recur throughout the year.

HEAD BANGING Exhibited by autistic, schizophrenic, or even reasonably normal children during temper tantrums. Can be a banging of the head against the floor or a wall or even hitting the head with an object. Understood psychoanalytically to be a means of assuring bodily integrity and realness when the child feels insufficiently attended.

HEARING, COLOR The hearing of particular sounds, or musical notes can produce color images for the subject. This phenomenon has been observed in high-IQ gifted individuals, outside any psychopathological diagnosis, and also observed in schizophrenic patients. Although not frequently encountered, this phenomenon is also not terribly rare.

HEBEPHRENIA Considered during most of the twentieth century in the psychiatric diagnostic nomenclature as one of the four basic types of schizophrenia. (The others were identified as the simple type, the catatonic type, and the paranoid type). This disorder is usually observed in onset before adulthood. The syndrome consists, in part, of delusions, severe cognitive dissembling, bizarre identity concerns, and emotional lability. A cardinal diagnostic key is the behavior of silliness and inappropriate laughter. See Schizophrenia.

HEDONISM The seeking of pleasure as a high-value characteristic of the personality. In contrast, the anhedonic state reflects the personality organization and manifest behavior of an individual in whom there seems an absence of any drive toward pleasure or toward seeking pleasure sources.

HERMAPHRODISM, PSYCHICAL Adler's phrase for the person's psychic organization in which the individual strives to gain the ascendancy over inferiority feelings. It is a compensatory attempt at achieving security through self-assurance as well as a typical Adlerian struggle for identity between the masculine and feminine orientation of the person.

HETEROEROTISM The cathectic libidinal investment in the opposite sex.

HIPPOCRATES (BC 460–370). Ancient Greek physician considered the father of medicine. Referred to temperaments of choleric and sanguine as a prelude to creating a typology classification. Considered the first classifier and utilized a model of humors and organs to account for personality. Suggested four humors of the body, from which, through imbalance, disease could result.

Humors	*Organ*	*Qualities*	*Temperament*
Blood	Heart	Heat	Sanguine
Phlegm	Brain	Dryness	Phlegmatic
Yellow bile	Liver	Moisture	Choleric
Black bile	Spleen	Cold	Melancholic

Cure rested in the administration of the quality opposite to that of the deficient humors. Among the many psychopathological states Hippocrates referred to were depression, suicide, delirium, and paranoia.

HOARDING Obsessive collecting. The objects collected need not be of any material value to the subject, although they will always be of psychic value. In extreme form, hoarding is a schizophrenic preoccupation and, in this pathological state, usually implies the prediction of further deterioration. Psychoanalytically related to the anal psychosexual phase. In Fromm's theory of character, the hoarding type is someone who does not feel he will ever get what he wants, finding it difficult, moreover, to engage in subject-object relationships. The hoarding is therefore an attempt to symbolically gain gratification with material objects, instead of person-to-person contact, along with containing the infrastructural components of symptom formation. See Symptom.

HOLDING ENVIRONMENT See Winnicott, D. W.

HOLIDAY SYNDROME The period between Thanksgiving and New Years Day sees a significant increase in psychiatric hospitalizations and suicides presumably resulting from repressed rage and a corresponding upsurge of anxiety and depression. Theoretically attributed to a reconstitution of early nuclear family unfulfilled wishes and trauma.

HOLISM Generally underpinning the Gestalt school of thought in which not only is the sum greater than its parts but also different from its parts. See Gestalt psychology.

HOMEOPATHIC PRINCIPLE Ernest Jones's notion that the identification of a repressed emotion will tend to lift the symptom. See Symptom.

HOMEOSTASIS Maintaining the balance of a system as in general systems theory. It is a calibration of stability. In personality theory, homeostasis refers to the balance of personality forces in the absence of destabilizing emotions such as terror, rage, or anxiety. In psychoanalytic thinking, homeostasis is the result of tension kept at a constant.

HOMESICKNESS In extreme form usually appears in persons who would be considered dependent, and who therefore wish for and seek to reconstitute the dependency constellation with the person(s) upon whom they have relied.

HOMEWORK Tasks to be done between cognitive behavior therapy or REBT sessions that have been collaboratively designed by client and therapist. They can be cognitive, emotive, or behavioral and may include reading assignments, relaxation, assertiveness practice, or maintaining logs of thoughts, feelings, and behavior. Also called self-help assignments.

HOMOLOGY The highest correlation between character and behavior.

HOMOPHOBIA Aversive reaction to individuals who are homosexual.

HOMOSEXUAL PANIC A severe panic or anxiety, involving, for example, a projection by the subject that another person of the same sex is being seductive with real intention of sexual contact. The projection, of course, reveals the latent homosexual urges of this selfsame subject. Clinically, acute depressive episodes or even schizophrenic decompensation can occur as a result of such panic, because this kind of latent homosexual impulse is in conflict with the extreme internalized prohibition against such an urge. This is especially the case in those individuals who have behaved in a heterosexual manner throughout their lives. At some trauma point, latent homosexual feelings can feel like impulses threatening to gain advantage and transcend internal controls and / or behavioral inhibitions. What is known as homosexual panic then becomes evident, and the subject is overcome with extreme tension and disabling anxiety.

HORIZON OF EXPERIENCE In the intersubjective theoretical lexicon this refers to the fluid, context-embedded boundary between conscious and unconscious.

HORNEY, KAREN (1885–1952). European-born American psychiatrist who promoted an approach in psychoanalysis that, in contrast to the biological underpinnings of Freudian psychoanalysis, stresses acculturation of attitudes in the development of neurosis. To Horney, the concept of basic anxiety and the person's need for a sense of safety are the salient vectors of her position regarding the dynamics of psychopathology. There are three types of personalities that comprise a typology in which she proposes criteria for each configuration:

The self-effacing type—movement toward people; the drive toward securing safety through compliance.

The expansive type—movement against people; relationships are seen as existing within an unending hostile struggle; to relieve anxiety and helplessness and achieve superiority, this type uses domineering and controlling measures; the strategy such a person uses is to manipulate in order to gain power and avoid weakness.

The resigned type—movement away from people; the motive here is to gain a sense of safety by arranging tactics to ensure emotional distance from people; such a person is determined to develop self-sufficiency and independence from others and can usually be found leading a withdrawn, isolated existence.

HOT COGNITION In cognitive behavior therapy, intense emotional reactions to new insights about oneself, others, or other situations. See Cold cognition.

HOUSE-TREE-PERSON TEST (HTP). A test developed in the mid twentieth century for the purpose of seeing an emotional / psychological X-ray of the child's inner life. Used with children over the age of three. The subject is asked to draw a house, a tree, and a person on separate sheets of blank paper; the psychologist draws implications regarding personality and family life from the drawings. At times the house-tree-person combination is drawn on a single sheet of paper. The test is also utilized to gauge brain damage or neurological involvement. Questions can be asked of the child, such as: "Is it a happy house?" or, "What is the child feeling?" In this way, as a projective device, the psychologist can elicit significant psychodynamic information regarding the nature of family conflict as well as a diagnostic assessment that can point to disturbing issues that may be affecting the child.

HUMANISTIC PSYCHOLOGY A field of psychology stressing a person's potential (as in Maslow's self-actualization). This humanistic tradition is a substantial break from the reductionistic Freudian tradition and is influenced by sources such as the work of Carl Rogers, the human potential movement, as well as concepts derived from existential psychology.

HYPERACTIVITY See Attention deficit/hyperactivity disorder. (ADHD).

HYPERKINETIC IMPULSE DISORDER This is more or less synonymous with attention deficit disorder.

HYPERSEXUALITY Abnormally increased sexual excitation and compulsive acting out of an obsessive focus on sex. For other than physiologic explanations, hypersexuality is usually attributed to compensatory needs designed by the person to validate the self. It is also seen as the ever present search for narcissistic gratification that continues to be reinforced and fortified by such compulsive sex searching and conquest. As a symptom it may refer to repressed anger regarding a pronounced sense of self-doubt.

HYPERSOMNOLENCE Excessive sleep. See Sleep disorders.

HYPERTENSION High blood pressure, considered as possibly the result of emotional/psychological tensions based upon intense competitiveness, intense wishfulness, ubiquitous underlying anger, as well as aggressive posturing that is always threatening to surface and that the person also then tries to suppress—not always with success. The stress of trying to manage this underlying anger becomes the main culprit in the aggregate pressure on the personality. Such individuals are also referred to as Type A personalities based upon obsessive striving, an excessive work ethic, and a relentless quest to satisfy wishes.

HYPERVENTILATION Rapid or shallow breathing that produces light-headedness, dizziness, sweating, and faintness. Generally caused by anxiety or underlying conflict in which anger is being suppressed. Also referred to as hyperventilation syndrome.

HYPNAGOGIC Referring to hypnoticlike sleep as in the state of the hypnagogic hallucination. See Hallucination; Narcolepsy.

HYPNAGOGIC HALLUCINATION See Hallucination; Narcolepsy.

HYPNOANALYSIS Also referred to as hypnotherapy. A technique of hypnosis utilized in psychotherapy to aid in the working through of a patient's resistance. The subject's attention is misdirected so that the suggestion by the hypnotherapist can be applied.

HYPNOGENIC ZONE See Zone, erogenous.

HYPNOSIS An altered state of consciousness promoted by the hypnotist's suggestion. Becomes more successfully applied to persons who are highly suggestible. Such suggestible types fall within the hysteric cluster of diagnostic entities. The more distant the diagnosis from the hysterical type, the more difficult it is for the hypnotic trance to take—for example, in the obsessive or guarded paranoid states.

HYPOCHONDRIASIS In the *DSM* nomenclature, considered to be a somatoform disorder in which the person becomes focused and overconcerned with the slightest indication of an ache, or pain, or some other unusual bodily experience. Frequently enough, the person so inclined, is instantly fearful of some deadly implication, often focusing on cancer or heart disease. Some psychoanalysts consider the hypochondriacal concern to reflect a depressive equivalent as well as representing narcissistic engagement, along with a corresponding reduction of interest in others. Another hypothesis that has been presented suggests that such a person harbors angry feelings toward some key past (historical) figure and searches for current transferential figures that could be used to reinforce underlying anger and, therefore, the hypochondriacal preoccupation.

HYPOKINESIS Slowed movements usually seen in depressed individuals.

HYPOMANIA Seen in individuals who are not quite manic, yet visibly excited, overtalking, impatient, and irrepressible.

HYPOSOMNIA Sleeping significantly less than a normal amount.

HYSTERIA One who is fearful or easily emotionally upset and therefore can lose control. Originally meant to reflect problems of women. Usually fused with the disposition of a hysterical personality, which has become the general reference of behavior and attitudes that are influenced by either direct or indirect suggestion. Thus suggestibility is the salient characteristic of the hysteric, along with dependency features that are also prominent. Further, hysteria also contains historical implications regarding the conversion reactions seen frequently in the nineteenth century, such as paralysis of limbs, as in the phrase *hysterical paralysis.* More recently, the diagnostic reference of hysteria has been associated with anxiety reaction or anxiety hysteria. Other considerations of the hysteric include *la belle indifference* formulated by Janet, designed to express the person's indifference. This indifference is of course related to the element of narcissism within the primitive fabric of the hysterical personality. Other examples of hysterical symptoms can include dissociated elements such as fugue, amnesia, or even trance behavior. The hysterical personality is also one in which sexuality can become flagrant and sexual variants such as seductive behavior are frequently typical. Emotional lability is also evident. In psychoanalytic terms, secondary gain of the conversion or dissociative state means that such a person gains some attention or concern from others with respect to the hysteric-seeming dysfunction. In the *DSM* nomenclature, the hysterical personality is also referred to as the histrionic personality.

HYSTERICAL PSYCHOSIS Under extreme pressure, conflict, or trauma, the hysterical personality can become an acute psychotic one. The psychotic symptoms will usually be short-lived, and prognosis is considered good. Under such conditions, when the personality decompensates and psychotic symptoms appear, these will usually be in the form of delusions and / or hallucinations.

HYSTEROGENIC ZONE See Zone, erogenous.

I

IATROGENY A concept accounting for the suggestibility of a person, so that, to varying degrees, the person's estimation of self becomes negatively affected. For example, the person can develop any number of neurotic hysterical symptoms based on what someone might say. Such a person might even begin to incubate a psychotic belief system, in response to the opinion of another as well.

IBs (IRRATIONAL BELIEFS) In rational emotive behavior therapy, these evaluative cognitions cause emotional disturbance and interfere with people's effectiveness in pursuing their goals. Albert Ellis identified three core irrational beliefs or philosophies that people hold:

1. I must do outstandingly well and be approved by others and, if not, I'm inadequate.
2. Other people must treat me well; if not, they are bad and should be punished.
3. Conditions of life must be comfortable and provide me with what I want, or else I won't be able to stand it and life will be rotten.

See ABCDE.

I-BOUNDARY A Gestalt therapy concept defining one's parameters with respect to a host of variables in the person's life, including how the person interacts with respect to attitudes, behavior, and values.

ID An element of Freud's structural theory. This structural theory sets the model for the interaction of id-ego-superego. The id is located in the unconscious mind, and it is comprised of primary process material, unformed and intense. The superego conforms to the rules and regulations of culture and prohibitions against unlawful impulse behavior and also exists unconsciously. The conflict between the id and superego is generally mediated by the ego, which is characterized by secondary process—rationality. While the id is governed by the pleasure principle, the ego is governed by the reality principle. See Freud, Sigmund.

IDEA(S) OF REFERENCE Usually referred to in paranoid diagnoses as the person either inventing out of thin air or taking what is being said by others and applying it to the self in some delusional idiosyncratic manner, that is to say, referring it to the self even when the other person did not intend it that way.

IDEALIZATION Psychoanalytic theory understands idealization as the attribution to another so-called adored figure of qualities to be admired—even worshipped. It is the ostensible transfer of love or libido to the loved object. Yet the idealization is also different from adoration insofar as it is considered a defense against ambivalence—thereby neutralizing the negative part of the ambivalence. Hence the defense of splitting occurs so that the idealized object can be divided into good and bad: the good is focused upon consciously, while the bad is denied. Thus the idealization does not lead solely to worship of the object, as much as it actually seems to imply a subservience to the object. Idealization in the Kohutian sense also refers to selfobject functions. See Selfobject functions.

IDEALIZED SELF A compensatory attempt to elevate the conception and persona of the self based upon a prototypic idealized image. Originally coined by Karen Horney.

IDEATION Thinking, forming ideas. Used clinically to assess a person's diagnostic condition—especially with reference to psychotic or schizophrenic thinking.

IDÉE FIXE One of the three pathological notions transformed into delusions:

The idée fixe—the person's insistence upon an idea (delusion), despite obvious evidence to the contrary.

The imperative idea—an obsession the person cannot shake, even though it is in fact seen by the subject to be inappropriate.

The autochthonous idea—based on a paranoid reference in which the force of the idea is sensed and believed as coming from an outside power or influence.

IDENTIFICATION Internalizing the attitudes and social orientation of an idealized mentoring figure. In the nature of enduring personality trait patterns, identification then becomes indispensable to the imprinting of etched traits. When such identifications are established, the person then calibrates emotions and tensions by internal rather than by external constraints. Controls are then reflexively implemented because of such implicit gyroscopic attitudes. Since identification is axiomatic, it occurs by example rather than instruction. The folklore adages "Like father, like son" and "The apple doesn't fall far from the tree" are based upon such automatic identification phenomena. Along with the defenses of internalization, splitting, symbolization, and turning against the self, identification is considered in the context of enduring personality trait formation. In contrast, the emotion defenses, or ego defenses of repression, denial, or reaction formation are designed to manage transitory emotional reactions and also double in their function as supports in the formation of the personality trait system. Identification has at least four different facets. These are

primary identification—undifferentiation of the infant from the mother;
secondary identification—the phase of differentiation from the object;
projective identification—imagining access to the mind of another that generates the feeling of control;
introjective identification—identifying with the introjected object as though the object is inside the subject.

IDENTIFICATION, PROJECTIVE See Projective identification.
IDENTIFICATION WITH THE SYMPTOM See Traversal of fantasy.
IDENTIFIED PATIENT That person in the family who is focused upon as the one with the problem. At times the identified patient may be the one who is ostensibly the problem person, but someone other may be the actual troubled one or the one creating the difficulty.
IDENTITY A person's self-image.
IDENTITY, EGO Refers to one's sense of self.
IDENTITY CRISIS Loss of one's sense of self. Clinically seen during anxiety crises, for example, a person during a

homosexual panic who has previously tried to identify as heterosexual.

IDENTITY DIFFUSION Chaotic moments in the sense of self, whereby the person experiences so-called split off parts of the self. Usually a diagnostic indication of borderline personality experience.

IDIOPATHIC Referring to a disease or psychopathology where the source or etiology of the disorder is unknown.

IDIOT Archaic term usually meaning retarded.

IDIOT SAVANT Historically considered to be a condition of mental deficiency along with special and even genius ability in particular areas of proficiency.

ID RESISTANCE See Resistance.

ILLUSION An inappropriate response to an external stimulus, as in misinterpreting something that is there. When the external stimulus is absent and the same response is made, the definition of such experience is termed a hallucination. Illusion is an important concept for Winnicott insofar as illusion, in the nonpejorative sense, reflects the point of congruence between the infants wish, on the one hand, and the mother's fulfillment of the wish, on the other. Contributors to the literature on illusion include Baumeister, Bettelheim, S. Freud, J. McDougall, Modell, Shor, Teitelbaum, Wheelis, Winnicott.

IMAGE, BODY One's concept of one's physical entity. Usually underestimated in importance with respect to one's psychological development. For example, if early in life, one is obese, but then later on trims down, nevertheless, despite the new appearance, the original obese body image is difficult to forget, and thus the original sense of imperfection becomes difficult to dislodge.

IMAGERY, HYPNAGOGIC A "twilight" phenomenon. This is a hypersensation of memory occurring when one is entering sleep, hypnopompic when waking. See Narcolepsy.

IMAGERY TECHNIQUE Frequently used in behavior therapy and cognitive behavior involving the client's imagining emotionally arousing scenes in combination with relaxation and / or cognitive restructuring.

IMAGO Meaning an image of early nuclear family members who remain etched in the unconscious.

IMBECILE Archaic term for retardation.

IMPLICIT RELATIONAL KNOWING Coined by Karlen Lyons-Ruth and the Boston Process of Change Group, based on neuropsychological research. Implicit relational knowing recognizes the procedural implicit communications between two people, patient and therapist, that occur on a nonconscious level. It informs communication and interpretation.

IMPOTENCE Male sexual dysfunction, in contrast to female sexual dysfunction (termed frigidity). In both cases libido becomes attenuated, so that, in men, variations of erectile dysfunction is symptomatic and, in women, vaginismus (tightening and closing of the vaginal muscles) or variations of nonorgasmic sexual functioning, is symptomatic.

IMPULSE Usually defined as a tendency to respond to a stimulus with a note of preemption. The term has been usurped as the psychoanalytic equivalent of instinct and is clinically assessed in the personality in conjunction with the person's ability to utilize controlling mechanisms—as in impulse versus control. Used synonymously with *drive.*

IMPULSE DISORDER Referring to attention deficit behavior, borderline symptoms, or psychopathic behavior. Clinically, the essence of impulse disorders concerns the issue of acting out.

IMPULSIVE In a clinical sense, refers to behavior that is mindless and reflects poor judgment or even absence of judgment—as in spur-of-the-moment reactions that usually result in negative outcomes.

INADEQUATE PERSONALITY In early diagnostic nomenclature, refers to individuals who underrespond in all spheres of functioning. This designation is no longer included in the most recent nomenclature, although it remains a useful clinical concept.

INATTENTION, SELECTIVE In psychoanalytic usage, seen as a convenient hysterical reaction in which the person utilizes the defense mechanism of denial in order to screen out unwanted information and then screen in information corresponding only to the subject's needs.

INCEST Sexual contact between family members, as, for example, in any oedipal sexual infraction.

INCIPIENT Used clinically to suggest that some psychopathological process exists, although only by inference and usually in the process of becoming—as in a yet uncrystallized state or even as an already formed latent construction.

INCOHERENCE Used generally when referring to diagnostic data, as in the confusion in speech observed during a schizophrenic episode.

INCORPORATION In psychoanalysis, refers to gratification of instinctual aims translated into ego gratifications and related to oral fantasies psychosexually. Somewhat synonymous with the term *identification,* as in the internalization of the stimulus. In emotion / personality theory, correlated to the emotion of acceptance.

INCUBUS Nightmare, more or less, and in past usage referring to the bad dream of a woman about a demon (man) conquering her sexually.

INDIVIDUAL PSYCHOLOGY The theoretical position of Alfred Adler, who parted from Freudian psychology to propose several tenets regarding the intrapersonal organization of the individual. Of the many concepts inherent in this Adlerian position, the striving for superiority and the sense of inferiority are two salient cornerstones of the theoretical network. See Adler, Alfred.

INDIVIDUATION Synonymous with the process of differentiation. In the work of Margaret Mahler, this object relations notion concerns the process of separation between mother and child when the child begins to differentiate itself from its primary caregiver. With reference to Jung, individuation relates to archetypes.

INDUCED PSYCHOTIC DISORDER Essentially a phenomenon of a folie à deux, shared, or double disturbance (usually psychotic and paranoid). When apparent, one sees such a phenomenon occurring, for example between mother and daughter, where the daughter begins to display symptoms that are the same as the mother's.

INDUCTION, DREAM Inducing a dream during hypnosis.

INELEGANT REBT (RATIONAL EMOTIVE BEHAVIOR THERAPY) In Ellis's REBT, a somewhat ineffectual form of disputing that involves questioning only a client's perceptions or attributions about an event (e.g., "My husband yelled at me; I infer that he doesn't love me."). Simply challenging this inference misses a deeper issue, such as "I must always do well and be completely loved by my husband, or I'm a failure." See Elegant REBT (Rational Emotive Behavior Therapy).

INFANTICIDE The murder of a child, usually by the mother, but also seen to be perpetrated by other nonmaternal figures. Historically, this phenomenon was identified as the murder of the infant immediately after birth and, in patriarchal societies, usually of female babies. Also seen to be of greater incidence in economically disadvantaged societies.

INFANTILE In clinical usage, most often referring to adult behavior that resembles pregenital behavior, thinking, and functioning. Similar to the general sense of immaturity.

INFANTILE SEXUALITY See Sexuality, infantile.

INFANTILE TRAUMA A trauma in infancy that is so intense that it becomes overwhelming and impossible for the infant to manage or master, ultimately leading to chronic tension and anxiety. Also referred to as primal trauma.

INFERIORITY A sense of inadequacy. The term was elevated to an important theoretical position by Alfred Adler in his individual psychology. Is also referred to by the lay public with respect to the phrase *inferiority complex.* See Complex, inferiority.

INHIBITION A psychoanalytic reference to the suppression of impulse.

INSANE The general usage for those individuals who are psychotic.

INSERTION THINKING Pressure of ideas. See Thought disorder.

INSOMNIA Difficulty in the process of sleep; usually either in falling asleep, awakenings during sleep, or early morning sleeplessness. In all three cases, daytime fatigue is experienced. Considered to be a dyssomnia in current *DSM* diagnostic terminology.

INSTINCT This is the basic mental energy in Freudian psychoanalysis. Instinct has a source, an object, and an aim. The source of the instinct is internal, its object is to express tension requiring gratification or satisfaction, and its aim is its gratification when it becomes experienced as a wish or desire. Instinct is also synonymous with the term *drive*. The inability of the instinct to find an object and, correspondingly, not to fulfill its aim always leads to frustration. The Freudian instincts were two at first: sexual (libido) and life preserving (ego), later changed to life (eros) and death (destrudo or thanatos) or translated clinically to libido and aggression. The aggressive instinct, if not directed outward, functions against the self in the form of regression—ultimately (unless deflected) bound to destroy the person. It also plays a role in Freud's theory of masochism. The life instinct, on the other hand, acts to preserve the self. Life's struggle is the constant equilibrium-disequilibrium of the two. Although instinct is considered an inborn drive to action, the psychoanalytic notion of instinct is also essentially an epigenetic one in which underlying tensions and impulses await their external environmental opportunities, which increase the possibility of expression. There are four basic vicissitudes of the instincts:

repression—use of defense mechanisms;
reversal—turning active to passive;
sublimation—transformation into symbolic form;
turning against the self—the self becomes the object.

INSTINCT REPRESENTATIVES Those derivative products, such as emotions and their attachment to ideas, that imply the presence of instincts and are their most visible representatives as well as they are of the pleasure principle.

INTEGRATED PSYCHOTHERAPY An eclectic approach to treatment that can include techniques from other approaches and are tailored for the particular patient.

INTELLIGENCE The ability to understand all sorts of relationships as well as ratios of these relationships with respect to a wide variety of categories and venues. These include verbal as well as nonverbal challenges. A sample of test construction psychologists in the development of measurement of intelligence have included Ammons, Spearman, Thorndike, Tolman, Wechsler. See Emotional intelligence.

INTELLIGENCE QUOTIENT (IQ) The score derived from an intelligence test. On the Wechsler scales, for example, 100 is considered normal (with a range of 90–110). The higher the score, the higher the IQ.

INTENTIONAL FORGETTING Essentially referring to repression related to material the subject didn't want to remember.

INTERMEDIATE BELIEFS In cognitive behavior therapy these are acquired beliefs that are similar to the superego injunctions of "shoulds" and "oughts." These beliefs include so-called hunches about what is best for the self and are not as entrenched as those of the core beliefs. Intermediate beliefs are frequently about pain and how to control it and are positioned between core beliefs and automatic thoughts (images existing alongside our conscious thoughts).

INTERMITTENT EXPLOSIVE DISORDER (IED) In the *DSM* nomenclature, considered an impulse-control disorder. This means that from time to time the subject erupts with anger and aggression and can even be assaultive. Such individuals are said to be characterized with a so-called thin stimulus barrier. See Thin stimulus barrier.

INTERNAL OBJECT See Object, internal.

INTERNAL SABOTEUR Related to Fairbairn's parsing of the antilibidinal ego that becomes an introduction to the development of superego. Also related to the rejecting object. The internal saboteur was a theoretical precursor of the rejecting object. It is always assaultive and retaliatory toward the self, as opposed to a higher-level superego that depends on the development of symbolic representations. It can be visceral and not necessarily verbal or visual.

INTERNALIZATION External objects that become etched in the psyche through the process of incorporating them, insofar as these are symbolic integrated representations.

INTERPERSONAL In addition to meaning the relation between people, this term also refers to Harry Stack Sullivan's theoretical position regarding the etiology of psychopathology based upon disturbed interpersonal relationships.

INTERPERSONAL PSYCHOTHERAPY A therapy seeking to denote the dynamic interplay of patient and therapist, with an eye toward reaching a catharsis through the working out of maladaptive patterns. Influenced by Sullivan and expected to be a shorter-term psychotherapy. Also influenced by Levenson and Klerman, who developed techniques in the here-and-now analysis of the patient within a social context. See Klerman, Gerald; Sullivan, Harry Stack.

INTERSUBJECTIVE COMMONALITY (COMMUNICATION) According to Schore, and in the domain of neuropsychoanalysis, in both the infant-mother and patient-therapist attachment relationships effective psychobiological transactions of unconscious affect involve right brain communications of facial expression, prosody, and gesture.

INTERSUBJECTIVE DISJUNCTIONS In intersubjectivity theory, when unconscious, these contribute to a therapeutic impasse, because the therapist experiences a meaning different from the meaning organizing the patient's experience.

INTERSUBJECTIVITY THEORY Key concept in self psychology and relational psychoanalysis, developed by Stolorow, Atwood, Brandchaft, and Orange, of recognizing interacting subjective states in oneself as well as in another person. Mutually constituted experience in the therapeutic relationship means that events are understood from a contextual point of view. In fact, the intersubjective position is that the analyst and the patient can mutually shape the conscious and unconscious experience of the other. The major shift in the intersubjective understanding is from the primacy of drives to the primacy of affectivity, also referred to as contextualism. Contributors to the arena of intersubjective theory as well as practice include Benjamin, Buirski, Daphne, Haglund, Monroe, Shane, Socarides, Stern, Teicholz, Trop, and Yi. See Stolorow, Robert.

INTRAPSYCHIC Refers to the interaction of id-ego-superego.

INTROJECTION The incorporation into the mental apparatus (or psyche) of an image or object (person)—usually idealized (the introjected object)—the purpose of which is to approximate the desired sense of persona and to support the ego. Revised by Stolorow, Atwood, Brandchaft, and Orange, emphasized by Kernberg.

INTROVERSION OR INTROVERTED TYPE A concept utilized by Freud to suggest that libido has been withdrawn from the objective of achieving some goal in relation to an object. The concept however, is usually more associated with the work of Jung, in his introversion-extraversion contrast, which identifies personality types.

INTUITION Sensing something. Good intuition is seen as the knack for accurate empathy. Those therapists who consider themselves to be intuitive also consider this quality to be indispensable to the successful process of perceiving, understanding, and interpreting. Another way of seeing it is to consider intuition as the combination of a mentation, sensation, and feeling that, in an amorphous way, constitutes a yet uncrystallized knowing. Akin to Bollas's "unthought known."

INTUITIVE TYPE See Jung, Carl Gustav.

INVOLUTION Referring to a regression from mature functioning.

INVOLUTIONAL PARANOIA See Paranoia, involutional

INVOLUTIONAL PSYCHOSIS Synonymous with melancholia or agitated depression. The involutional period for women is from age forty to fifty-five, and for men fifty to sixty-five. Symptoms are usually in the category of depression, delusions, and obsessions. Emotions of dread and despair accompany such symptoms.

INWARD PICTURE Jung's conception of one's most valid picture of the self, referred to as "the true self."

IRRATIONAL BELIEFS (IBs) In REBT, these rigid, absolute, and illogical beliefs are at the core of most emotional disturbance and self-defeating behavior. The four irrational beliefs or processes involve

1. *awfulizing/catastrophizing* (AWF)—extreme or exaggerated evaluations of events as opposed to viewing them as unpleasant or inconvenient;
2. *demandingness* (DEM)—the tendency to substitute shoulds, oughts, and musts for preferences (e.g., my partner must love me);
3. *low frustration intolerance* (LFT)—The person's perceived inability to tolerate or survive the discomfort of a situation or event;
4. *global evaluation/self doubting* (GE/SD). Rating people as totally bad, as opposed to only rating their behavior.

See Ellis, Albert; Hot cognitions; IBs (Irrational beliefs); Rational Emotive Behavior Therapy (REBT).

IRRATIONALITY An important concept in diagnosis, acting out, and reality testing. It means unreasonable, inappropriate, and not in keeping with a normal, expected response to the stimulus that is presented. It is perhaps the pathological parallel to originality.

IRRITABLE BOWEL SYNDROME (IBS) Abdominal discomfort as well as bowel difficulties are seen to be, at least in part, a function of psychological factors related to anxiety and, likely, to repressed anger.

ISAKOWER PHENOMENON Coined by European psychoanalyst Otto Isakower (1899–1972). He identified various strange hallucinatorylike symptoms whereby individuals experience objects moving, or even spinning, hither and fro in space. Psychoanalytically, seen as a revival of being at the breast. Also, may be identified as a blank hallucination. See Hallucination.

ISOLATED MIND In intersubjective theory, the idea of the isolated mind contrasts the intersubjective with a contextualist psychoanalytic model. Rather than seeing relationships as coconstructed, the metapsychology of traditional psychoanalytic thinking is considered as treating relationships as though part of a one-person psychology. In contrast, relational theory sees relationships as coconstructed, with the contributions of each partner neither equal, symmetrical, nor similar.

ISOLATION OF AFFECT The separation of an emotion from a memory of a person or an event. Considered to be a defense mechanism mostly seen as part of the obsessional defense syndrome.

J

JACOBSON, EDITH (1897–1978). European psychoanalyst/ego psychologist who considered libidinous and aggressive drives to be fundamental and yet also posited that drives are influenced by the early caretaker (mother). The infant therefore was also seen as being influenced by inner object representations as well as by drives. In addition, Jacobson felt that the self, through the phenomenon of self-representation, can be acted upon by the drives as though it were an object. Deviations that occur at this point can lead to later psychopathology. Jacobson also contributed to the understanding of narcissistic, borderline, and depressive functioning and postulated that psychosis was a function of poor differentiation between subject and object. She also suggested that consistent frustration and disappointments during infancy would later lead to depression. In contrast, assimilation and balance of positive and negative feelings was considered to be healthy and to block the strong primitive drives of libido and aggression. Jacobson also differentiated ego from self, judging ego to be the key psychic structure, while attributing to the self the role of reflecting the total person. She also made significant alterations to the understanding of superego and even postulated that certain defenses, rather than being relegated to ego function, are instead a service of and governed by the superego. Jacobson influenced Kohut and Kernberg.

JANET, PIERRE French psychiatrist (1842–1910). Predating Freud, Janet proposed unconscious processes associated with phenomena of dissociation.

JANOV, ARTHUR American psychologist (1924–). Created an experiential psychotherapy. See Primal therapy.

JEALOUSY The Freudian position on jealousy is that it must be connected to the experience of the lost love object. A person experiencing jealousy feels such a loss as a blow to self-esteem and a narcissistic injury. In the extreme case, jealousy can lead to violence toward the object of hatred (who has come to possess the loved object). In psychoanalysis, jealousy is understood as a derivative drama of the oedipal triangle. Freud postulated that pathological jealousy is related to paranoia and homosexuality. Jealousy always contains anger.

JOHARI WINDOW Developed by Luft and Ingham to assess insight individuals have in communication with others. An imaginary window with four panes comprises the self-knowledge parameter. These include panes that are

open—information is known to both people;
blind—information is known only to the other person;
hidden—information is known only to the subject;
unknown—information is not known to either person.

JORDAN, CATHLEEN (1947–). Professor of social work, University of Texas. Author of volumes on clinical assessment and family therapy. Former director, University of Texas doctoral program. Member, editorial board, *Dictionary of Psychopathology.*

JUDGMENT A term used in psychology to assess one's index of appropriateness. On intelligence tests, and on projective tests, the psychologist is always interested in the level and nature of the person's judgment.

JUNG, CARL GUSTAV (1875–1961). Swiss psychiatrist. One of Freud's earliest disciples, who split with Freud to develop his own school of psychoanalysis called analytic psychology. Jung formulated the idea of archetypes as well as of the collective unconscious and developed a broad theory of symbols. Among the early psychoanalysts, Jung is considered by many to be the mystic, but, aside from Freud, arguably the most influential. Popularized notion of types:

Introversion—more interested in the self.
Extraversion—more interested in the object.

Functional types postulated by Jung:

Rational Class of Functional Types

The feeling type—attitudes governed by feelings.

The thinking type—person's behavior is governed by reflection.

Irrational Class of Functional Types

The intuitive type—called the irrational one, because such a person's perceptions and interpretations are based on scant evidence, along with an overreliance on incidental data. A superperceptive person.

The sensational type—sensation equals perception, as in sense perception. Such perception is conscious and dominant over emotion and cognition, although not necessarily dominant with respect to intuition. This sort of person focuses on the enjoyment of sensation and enjoyment generally.

Mental Levels

A Jungian concept that, by implication, elevates the notion of cultural, historical, and, perhaps, even racial consciousness. Jung divides such levels into

consciousness—contains the persona or mask the person displays to the world;

unconscious—suppressed and forgotten memories;

collective unconscious—archetypical psychic contents relevant to society in its entirety.

Jung's idea of function includes

function, archaic—notion of regression into the unconscious whereby an absent libido creates a chaotic and archaic inner life;

function engram—a symbol derived from a general sense of the collective unconscious, described as emanating from the psyche of society itself or even the race; Jung's conception of categories was based on the rather fallacious notion that "race" or "society" represented strictly pure homogeneous groupings, which assumption largely accounted for crazed Nazi heredity theorists adopting the Jungian understanding of human nature;

function type—overall consideration of types: thinking, feeling, intuition, and sensation.

K

KARDINER, ABRAHAM (1891–1981). American psychoanalyst/anthropologist. One of the early psychoanalytic pioneers. Considered to be a cultural psychoanalyst as well. He was interested in the cross-cultural psychodynamic that he termed psychological anthropology. His system was based upon three related concepts that underpinned the individual's requirement to become competent in the culture:

Primary institutions—includes child-rearing responsibilities such as feeding or weaning infants;
Secondary institutions—includes societal structures such as schools and economic means of production;
Personality structures—formed by primary institutions and projected onto societal institutions.

KAVALER-ADLER, SUSAN (1950–). American psychologist/psychoanalyst. Object relations theorist. Authored volumes in the domains of developmental mourning and psychic change, creativity, the demon lover complex, and erotic transference in interaction with developmental mourning. Provided psychobiographies of women writers. Founder of the Object Relations Institute for Psychotherapy and Psychoanalysis. Member, editorial board, *Dictionary of Psychopathology.*

KELLERMAN, HENRY (1938–). American psychologist/psychoanalyst. Author and editor. Formulated understanding of the infrastructure of psychological symptom formation. Connected the personality system to Plutchik's psychoevolutionary theory of emotion and developed a theory of the nightmare as it is correlated to the various facets of personality. Authored volumes on psychopathology and differential diagnosis, special symptom disorders, psychodiagnostics, group theory, emotions and personality, and the psychoanalysis of symptoms. Author, *Dictionary of Psychopathology*. See Symptom.

KERNBERG, OTTO (1928–). Austrian-born and Chilean-educated psychiatrist-psychoanalyst. Known for his formulations of borderline and narcissistic pathologies. Utilizes Freudian metapsychology, but is more aligned with object-relations psychology within an ego psychology framework. According to Kernberg, mother-child interaction determines the relative success of maturation. His psychic apparatus permits object relations conceptions to prevail over Freudian drive theory. Kernberg proposes that in borderline and narcissistic pathologies metabolism (maturing by assimilating earlier relating patterns) is insufficiently developed. Thus, acting out dominates the personality.

Three basic kinds of internalization occur during normal development:

Ego identity—stable view of objects and integrated sense of self.

Identification—self and object are understood, symbolized, and not threatening.

Introjection—primitive, undifferentiated sense of self is internalized.

Primitive Defenses

devaluation—minimizing the object to support the narcissistic warding off of the inadequate internal self that would threaten mortification and the breakdown of the false grandiose self structure.

idealization—controls latent hostility and mistrust and reflects a paranoid projection, or a loving one, depending on the diagnosis.

projective identification—putting into the object, the repudiated part of the self; it is not a simple cognitive projection; the other who is projected onto and provoked is a living external presence.

splitting—parsing good and bad parts of self and object representations.

KEY QUESTION A technique designed by Alfred Adler that acts as a trigger, somewhat resembling a Socratic question, to elicit a response that would imply the patient's attitude about existing pathology.

KINESICS The psychology of movement as it relates to styles of communication.

Kinesthetic hallucination—the sense of something in motion where nothing is there, as in the sense of the presence of a phantom limb. Analogous to blank hallucination.
Kinesthetic sensation—the person's sense of space around the body and the relationship-distance to others.

KINSEY, ALFRED CHARLES (1894–1956). American biologist known for his extensive studies and surveys of sexuality. Credited for relaxing the mores of sexual behavior by demonstrating the widespread variety of sexual practices.

KLEBENBLEIBEN A form of associative disturbance seen in schizophrenic patients in which perseveration (repeating) occurs, but in the form of shaping and reshaping the same thought from different angles.

KLEIN, MELANIE (1882–1960). A British child psychoanalyst who developed an object relations theory and defined basic developmental "positions," such as the paranoid, schizoid, and depressive, that, when identified, reveal personality information regarding maturational processes and normal and abnormal development. Ego development is seen to be replete with introjections and projections of objects; unlike Freud's system of psychosexual stages, Klein sees the crux of development occurring in the first year of life. Key derivatives are envy and aggression. Her phenomenology of two psychic positions define development and self integration. She enumerates "positions" of the infant's experience:

- *paranoid/schizoid position*—a most primitive level of development, during the first three months of life, in which the infant projects disowned parts of the self. The basic anxiety here is that persecutory objects—the bad ones—will invade the self. Here the ego is paranoid, but also schizoid, insofar as bad objects are projected, and good ones protected. Thus the infant protects itself from its own death instinct by projecting aggression in order to neutralize this external threat. Part of this process includes the appearance of "introjection," and "splitting," which basically establishes the model for the internalization of the good and bad object.

- *depressive position*—at about six months to two years, negative or painful aspects of the self can be contained and the infant can have empathy for the self and the other. Guilt and loss are reasonably tolerated, and even ambivalence toward the love object can be consciously experienced. Therefore, the mother is seen more in a whole sense. Yet, with an anxiety that seems psychologically palpable, the apprehension exists that the mother may be destroyed by the death instinct. Mourning of loss is a critical clinical and developmental process. In general, the defensive mechanics of splitting, and the projective mechanisms, are two of the salient levers in Kleinian epistemology that address her "positions." Only in the depressive position is the subjectivity of the self experienced and therefore empathy for another's subjectivity can be realized. The chief threat is object loss.

KLEPTOMANIA A compulsive desire to steal, an acting out. Psychoanalysts offer the explanation that the stealing is a condensed symbolic act of reempowerment for the person's perceived lack of power. Frequently the stealing will be linked to someone who is in a position considered by the subject to be better, higher, or more important. Because of this, anger lurks. Psychoanalytically related to wishes of oedipal conquest—stealing the other.

KLERMAN, GERALD (1929–1992). American psychiatrist. Known for his formulation of interpersonal therapy in which the treatment consists of events of the "here and now." Deeper psychoanalytic precepts are eschewed in favor of discussions of problems within a social context. Contributor to theory and research on depression and schizophrenia.

KLINE, NATHAN S. (1917–1983). American psychiatrist. Pioneer in the biochemical treatment of depression. Founded the Nathan S. Kline Institute for Psychiatric Research.

KLOPFER, BRUNO (1900–1971). European-born American psychologist influential in projective psychology and personality testing. Contributed mightily to the popularity of the Rorschach as the major projective instrument of the test battery. Coauthored classic two-volume Rorschach text with Mary Ainsworth, Robert Holt, and Walter Klopfer. See Rorschach Test.

KOHUT, HEINZ (1913–1981). Viennese psychiatrist/psychoanalyst who trained in the United States. He developed self psychology. Kohut reconceptualized the understanding of narcissistic disorders, focusing on the centrality of the sense of self and its cohesion. He created a new lexicon to describe phenomena of early development. Post-Kohutian thinking influenced by psychoanalytic self psychology can roughly be divided into three new traditions:

Intersubjective systems—primarily conceived and developed by Stolorow, Atwood, Brandchaft, and Orange.

Motivational systems—primarily conceived and developed by Joseph Lichtenberg, and elaborated by Lichternberg, Lachmann, and Fosshage.

Dyadic mutual regulation system—co-creation of the interaction between infant and caretaker, relevant to adult treatment. Developed by Abend, Tronick and Beebe and Lachmann.

A sample of other contemporary contributors to the investigation into and expansion of self-psychology include Bacal, Buirski, Goldberg, Ornstein, Stern, Wallerstein, Wolfe. See Intersubjectivity theory; Self psychology.

KORSAKOFF ALCOHOLIC PSYCHOSIS Equivalent to chronic alcoholic delirium, in which a wide variety of cognitive functions become impaired.

KRAEPELIN, EMIL (1856–1926). European psychiatrist who was influential in the development of personality typologies as well as making the earliest distinction between manic-depressive psychosis and schizophrenia. Differentiated dementia praecox to include the following subtypes:

Catatonic—reference to immobility and explosiveness;
Hebephrenic—inappropriate reactions;

Mute and excited behavior—early reference to affective disorder;

Paranoid—delusions of persecution.

KRAFFT-EBING, RICHARD VON (1840–1903). European physician known as the first sexologist; espoused a hereditary degenerative theory of illness considered to be deviance.

KRETSCHMER, ERNST (1856–1926). European psychiatrist. Related physical type to personality type, initiating the field referred to as somatotyping or personality typing. His types were based upon two disorders—schizophrenia and manic-depressive psychosis. The schizophrenic type was labeled schizoid, and the manic-depressive cycloid. The schizoid was unsociable and reserved, while the cycloid was sociable and impulsive. His typology included references to temperament and physique:

The asthenic or leptosome type—was a person with an elongated body build who was of the schizoid side, aesthetic, and sensitive.

The athletic type—muscular; less likely to display psychopathology.

The pyknic type—was heavier, shorter, and broader in body type, and corresponded to the cycloid affective side.

KRIS, ERNST (1900–1957). European-born American psychoanalyst and art historian. Formulated concept of regression-in-the-service-of-the-ego as it also relates to sublimation. Closely associated with Freud and coedited Freud's *Collected Psychological Works.*

L

LA BELLE INDIFFERENCE In conversion hysteria, the person is seemingly indifferent to the symptom or signal anxiety. Not being alarmed. Seen also in schizophrenia.

LABILE Clinical instability characterized by dyscontrol of emotion.

LACAN, JACQUES-MARIE-EMIL (1901–1981). Influential French psychiatrist-psychoanalyst who shifted focus of psychoanalysis away from biology and physics to language and linguistic structure. Yet his is a return to Freud in contrast to the difference between Freud and ego psychology. Basically, Lacan posited that ego identity is a mosaic of identifications, with language the crucial variable in all of psychoanalysis. Identity variables include

the mirror stage—in the process of identification, this stage is one in which the child learns to see itself from outside of the self as a precursor to an internal identity.
the others—identification is constituted in the other—of the external world. You know yourself because of being different from the other;
the real, the imaginary, and the symbolic—elements of the psyche.

The person receives stimuli in "registers." There are three such registers.

The real register—equivalent to a Freudian primary process amorphous bombardment of stimuli as in experiencing but without interpretation or understanding. It is the world in a state of prelanguage and therefore it cannot be directly accessed. It can only be indirectly reached through the imaginary and symbolic registers.
The imaginary register—all of fantasy is included, but in the absence of a sense of the self. This is ego in the structural (not dynamic) sense of identity.
The symbolic register—where a sense of self is known when experience becomes infused within language structure. It is the ordering of the structure of language in which the symbolic automatically crystallizes.

LACHMANN, FRANK (1929–). American psychologist/psychoanalyst forging a meeting between self psychology and infant research. Collaborated with Beatrice Beebe, Joseph Lichtenberg, Robert Stolorow, and

James Fosshage. Authored volumes expanding self-psychology into such areas as aggression, humor, creativity, and perversion. Known also for his work in the supervision of the therapeutic process. Founding faculty of the Institute for the Study of Subjectivity. Member, editorial board, *Dictionary of Psychopathology.*

LACUNAE, SUPEREGO, Largely interpreted with acting-out personalities (such as psychopaths) to mean moral gaps. Such gaps are designed by the subject to undermine the object in order to reduce the difference in stature between object and self. Considered to represent contamination or pathology of the superego, which in psychoanalytic terms can also be seen as a "superego leak."

LAING, R. D. (1927–1989). Scottish psychiatrist who focused on the social/political underpinnings of psychopathology and was interested in the experience of psychosis. Popular in the radical 1960s. Philosophically, he was an existentialist who made a lasting impression with respect to the importance of an ethical stance in the treatment of psychiatric patients.

LALOPATHY Referring to speech disorders.

LANGUAGE, IRRELEVANT Seen in schizophrenic patients who will speak idiosyncratically so that some words or sentences have a meaning specific only to them.

LANGUAGE, METAPHORIC Use of images in language that can enhance creative expression. Also similar to irrelevant language insofar as the person may utilize images that are so idiosyncratic as to have meaning only to the person using it.

LATENCY A Freudian term used in the description of psychosexual development. In his psychosexual theory, Freud postulated the stages of oral, anal, phallic, and oedipal. The latency phase begins about the late oedipal stage—at about five years of age—and retains its character until about puberty. In the so-called normal or healthy latency phase of development, the child utilizes sublimation mechanisms to manage sexual and aggressive impulses so that these impulses remain moderated. In a modern society, the latency-age child focuses on schooling as the sublimated arena. In tribal societies, the focus is on apprenticeship learning of ritual requirements preparatory to initiation into membership in the tribe at puberty or adolescence.

LATENCY, SLEEP See Sleep latency.

LATENT Underlying, as in the psychoanalytic understanding of dreams. The latent actual meaning of a dream underlies the manifest or story line of the dream that the dreamer actually sees while dreaming or remembers after dreaming. In psychoanalysis the manifest dream is unfolded in order to mine the latent content of the dream by having the dreamer associate to the different elements of the manifest content of the dream; this is the latent dream from below, unraveled from the manifest dream from above. Also referred to in the therapeutic setting with reference to an underlying meaning of a patient's comments or gestures. Latent content is essentially concealed or dormant—not manifest.

LATENT DREAM See Dream theory, Freudian.

LAZARUS, ARNOLD ALLAN (1932–). South African–born American cognitive behavioral therapist who pioneered multimodal therapy, a unique assessment and treatment approach that deals with what is termed the BASIC ID (Behavior, Affect, Sensation, Imagery, Cognition: Interpersonal relationships and Drugs / Biology. See BASIC ID; Multimodal therapy.

LAZARUS, RICHARD (1922–2002). American psychologist. Pioneer of cognitive appraisal theory, in which emotion becomes a function of contextual appraisal. An avid researcher into the operation of emotion, Lazarus was interested in seeing how emotion and stress related to cognition. His is considered a cognitive phenomenological theory of emotion.

LD OR LEARNING DISABILITIES Referring generally to developmental problems that may not be due to brain or biological defects.

LEARNED HELPLESSNESS A risk factor for depression described by American psychologist Martin Seligman involving lack of motivation and sense of defeat in facing certain uncomfortable experiences over which the person perceives himself to have no control, when in fact they actually may have available options. See Seligman, Martin.

LEWIS, HELEN BLOCK (1913–1987). American psychologist/psychoanalyst known for theory and research. Author of volumes treating guilt and shame and the role of shame in symptom formation. See Shame.

LIBIDO Originally a Freudian term for sexual drive and later used in opposition to the aggressive drive. Libido also is a form of mental energy invested with object representations—creating the power of bonding in relationships. See Dopaminergic "seeking" system; Panksepp, Jaak.

LIBIDO MOBILITY A reference to the ability of the person to shift emotional investment or libidinous investment from one person to another. The psychoanalytic term for this investment is cathexis. See Cathexis.

LIBIDO STASIS Freud noted that when libido is not permitted its motor expression, tensions accumulate and one may grow overly sensitive to auditory sensations, becoming irritable, anxious, and even hypochondriacal.

LIBIDO THEORY Referring to the sexual drive.

LIFE-EVENT STRESS THEORY Individual signal events are considered more significant than typical continuous events as predictions for later functioning. See Continuity theory.

LIFE GOAL Adlerian concept referring to the overall issue of striving and realization of one's wishes. This compensatory operation is an implied ever present structural support that facilitates a relentless striving toward a goal, defending against any inferiority feelings or even pessimism.

LIFE PLAN Adler's point that the person will create a strategy of attitude and behavior that ultimately supports, reinforces, and fortifies the feeling of superiority. Psychoanalytically, the defense of denial and the presence of sufficient ego strength would be implicated in the person's ability to retain the necessary sense of self in the face of daily challenges—especially those that result in disappointment.

LIMB, PHANTOM A person's sense that a lost limb is still there. This mental representation usually follows the abrupt loss or removal of the limb by surgery, war, or accident.

LIMBIC SYSTEM According to Westen, in the domain of neuropsychoanalysis, the limbic system enables a conscious recognition in the other of qualities of the self that are unconsciously repudiated, which in psychodynamic terms is essentially defined as projective identification. In Klein's view, these disavowed feelings are projected to the analyst, resulting in the patient treating the analyst negatively, by which means the patient maintains a measure of control. Decisions are driven from the source limbic system by emotions that are correspondingly unconscious. Schore states that the limbic system derives subjective information as emotions that guide behavior, allowing the brain to adapt to a rapidly changing environment and organize new learning. See Thinking.

LINE, THE Separates reality from fantasy. Front of the line represents a reality-doing place where people implement activity toward the achievement of goals. Behind the line is a place of withdrawal, rumination, compensatory fantasy, and magical thinking. It is typical for all people to step behind the line several times during waking hours as a method of "taking a break—a breath." It is the undue time spent behind the line that signals withdrawal into fantasy, especially compensatory fantasy. See Withdrawal.

LINEHAN, MARCIA (1943–) American psychologist who has been instrumental in developing cognitive behavioral strategies and techniques for the treatment of a variety of psychopathological disorders. See Dialectical Behavioral Therapy (DBT).

LINGUISTIC-KINESIC METHOD With respect to disturbed behavior, a method of better understanding communicational disturbance, both verbal and nonverbal behavior.

LITTLE HANS A classic case treated by Freud of a little boy with a phobia about horses. Freud determined that the phobia was etiologically related to the boy's anger at his father and proposed castration anxiety and oedipal implications as part of his understanding of the case. The published case is entitled *An Analysis of a Phobia in a Five-Year-Old Boy.*

LOBOTOMY, PREFRONTAL Surgery of the frontal lobe originally popularized for the treatment of intractable aggression and performed widely in the 1940s and 1950s. Patients then became what is known as vegetative—that is, essentially losing interest in the color of emotion generally, not merely in the management or elimination of anger. Considered by many to be a vestige of medieval medicine.

LOEWALD, HANS (1906–1993). European-born American psychiatrist / psychoanalyst. Promoted understanding of pre-oedipal development and studied integrative experiences in the transference as a key to therapeutic working through.

LOGOTHERAPY An existential therapy based upon a search for meaning and related to spiritual or social issues, rather than strictly psychological considerations or biologically based assumptions. It strongly values the sense of responsibility possessed by individuals to resolve blocks to what is called the will to meaning.

LOVE In personality trait theory, love is the combination of acceptance and joy, minus any anger toward the love object. Love may also always contain a transferential element to some historical figure. Psychoanalytically, the swoon of love tends to anesthetize what, for the sake of metaphor, may be called the psychological immune system. In this way, the acceptance of the other (the graft of self and other) is not rejected. The love swoon, therefore, is a bonding mechanism, relating to "attachment theory" and ultimately to the work of Bowlby. A central issue of theology, empirically associated with, sequentially related to, responding to, or inextricably linked to forgiveness, guilt, fear of abandonment, anger, and even hate. See Neuropsychoanalysis of oedipal behavior.

LOVE, GENITAL A psychoanalytic concept meaning mature loving or mature relating.

LOVE, PREGENITAL Essentially the child's love toward the mother.

LOW FRUSTRATION TOLERANCE (LFT) Important concept identified by U.S. psychologist and founder of REBT

Albert Ellis, who viewed this process (also called discomfort disturbance or I-can't-stand-it-it is) as a major factor in self-pity, love neediness, addiction, anger, anxiety, compulsivity, procrastination, and other disorders. See Irrational beliefs.

LUNATIC Archaic term for one with a mental problem. Used synonymously with *insane.*

M

MCDOUGALL, JOYCE (1920–). French psychoanalyst. Her many contributions include investigations into the psychological and emotional vicissitudes of child development. Her seminal contributions are with patients suffering from psychophysiological symptoms as well as issues related to sexual identity and the perversions.

MCDOUGALL, WILLIAM (1871–1938). American psychiatrist whose contribution to the study of psychopathology focused on the classification of the emotions.

MACHOVER, KAREN (1902–1996). American psychologist who created the Machover Draw a Person projective test, a standard part of the projective test battery from which the psychologist can derive a rather significant profile of the personality. See Machover Draw a Person Test (DAP).

MACHOVER DRAW A PERSON TEST (DAP). This is a projective test where subjects are asked to draw a person on a blank sheet of paper. Results of the test regarding a host of personality features can be implied by various interpretations based on the kind of drawing made. The uncovering of such meanings was pioneered by the American psychologist Karen Machover. The test is generally referred to as the Machover Draw a Person Test. Examples of various elements of interpretation include

size of the figure—reference to self-esteem;

location of the figure on the page—reference to withdrawal or shyness versus narcissism or grandiosity are examples of meaning;

full face or profile of the figure—reference to possible paranoia;
nature of line quality—reference to possible anger or depression;
shading or no shading—reference to issue of anxiety;
focus and detail on sensory organs such as the eyes—possible reference to paranoia;
compartmentalization of body parts or not—reference to obsessional-compulsive state;
treatment of hands and feet—reference to passivity or assertion;
body axis distortion—possible indication of psychosis;
transparencies—indication of poor reality testing and possible psychosis;
line emphasis on wrists, ankles, and neck—possible reference to suicidal implications.

MCWILLIAMS, NANCY R. (1945–). American psychologist/psychoanalyst. Contributor to the arena of personality structure and diagnosis, feminist theory and psychoanalysis, as well as to the understanding of dissociative personality.

MADAM BUTTERFLY FANTASY The fantasy, reflecting the wish of the return of a loved one who has either died or disappeared.

MAGICAL THINKING Wishful thinking considered to be derivative, psychoanalytically, of the oral stage of psychosexual development. Tension regarding the person's aspirations are assuaged through fantasy. This is particularly true of the phenomenon of creating fantasy scenarios in which such aspirations are achieved. Magical thinking is diametrically opposite to real implementation activities directed eventually, and through effort, toward reaching one's goals. See Primitivization.

MAGIC HELPER Erich Fromm's phrase for describing the dependent personality whose main wish is to search for and find some authority with whom to relate. Thus the magic helper ensures the subject's protection and emotional sustenance.

MAHLER, MARGARET (1897–1985). European psychiatrist. Studied the child's world in the context of the mother-child dyad. This object relations study is connected to the domains of ego psychology and developmental psychoanalytic psychology and concerns the internalizations and introjections of early interpersonal contact—especially with the mother. Mahler's theory of ego and personality development consisted of a series of stages:

Autistic phase—earliest phase, in which the child cannot discriminate between self and mother and therefore strives to sustain a state of tensionless balance.

Symbiotic phase—second phase, in which separation between mother and child begins, and the mother is therefore gradually seen as the gratifying separate object—although joined to the self. It is during this phase that the child begins to regulate tension and to develop ego functions. Impairments in this symbiosis can result in psychotic reactions.

Separation / individuation phase—child senses self as separate, through a series of experiences reflecting differentiation, practicing, rapprochement, and self-identity.

Mahler contributed diagnostic clarification related to borderline pathology as this pathology derived from problems in the separation / individuation stage. She advanced the understanding and treatment of the borderline patient's defective sense of identity (including sexual confusion), as well as elaborating the faulty emotional regulation of such borderline functioning. Mahler also detailed a theory of normal development and enumerated the variables associated with anxiety and psychopathology generally.

MAIN'S SYNDROME Usually a pathology in which a female patient invites sympathy and concern from professional medical personnel by regaling these professionals with personal details of ostensible and continuous incestuous experiences. Observed by T. F. Maine in the mid 1950s.

MAINTENANCE LEVEL The particular dosage required to sustain a desired medication effect.

MALADJUSTMENT Clinically equivalent to the diagnosis of adult situational disorder, meaning poor adaptation including faulty judgment, immature functioning, and responding idiosyncratically rather than in a so-called normal fashion. Also equivalent to the concept of degree of disturbance and refers in a general sense to psychopathology.

MALAPROPISM Mistakenly sounded words because of similarity of sound to another word.

MALE ERECTILE DISORDER Difficulty of the male in having or sustaining an erection. Frequently seen in older men because of problems resulting from the aging process, but can be a psychological problem in younger men as well. See Sexual dysfunction.

MALEVOLENT TRANSFORMATION Sullivanian conception of paranoia in which a person constructs a perceived surrounding world replete with nothing but enemies.

MALIGNANT TREND Pointing toward the inexorable development of a chronically debilitating condition.

MALINGERING Feigning illness for some personal gain. In differential diagnostic psychology, malingerers are for the most part considered paranoid or psychopathic. They try to outsmart whatever observer is assessing them by logically calibrating their own behavior so that whatever illness is being feigned will not appear to be revealing any contraindication. In contrast, the hysterical personality will be ruled out as a malingerer because the hysteric can usually dispel with any symptom and at any time that another need becomes more important and therefore prevails, even in a way that defies logic. Such a person does not really care about the illogic of their particular behavior, whereas the malingerer cares a great deal about logic.

MANDALA A Jungian term referring to the unity of the self.

MANIA Characterized by euphoria, agitation, overactivity (called psychomotor overactivity), compulsive talking, the taking on of many projects simultaneously, impulsive behavior, elation, doing everything speedily, grandiosity, shifting of subject matter, distractibility, inability to sleep, flight of ideas. These represent a cluster of behaviors that characterize this sort of mood disorder. In diagnostic terminology mania usually refers to manic-depressive psychosis. Psychoanalytically, mania is thought to be a victory over the superego and a defense against depression—the depression resulting from a hostile superego.

MANIC-DEPRESSIVE PSYCHOSIS Affective psychosis in which manic and depressive episodes occur. See Bipolar disorder; Psychosis.

MANIC EPISODE A particular manic event characterized as acute and serious enough to warrant intervention.

MANNERISM Idiosyncratic behavior that seems overpersonalized and therefore not in keeping with conventional behavior.

MAO INHIBITORS Monoamine oxidase, a drug used for antidepressant treatment.

MARITAL THERAPY A type of psychotherapy focused on the marital couple, in which, in addition to examining each person's conflicts, the couple as a unit is primarily considered to be the patient. Thus there are three patients in marital therapy—each partner as well as the couple.

MARRIAGE, SANDBOX Euphemism for which partner will win the competition for becoming the one most mothered by the other.

MASCULINE PROTEST For both men and women this protest reflects a drive to negate the feminine role in whatever pejorative form it is seen. For Alfred Adler, it forms the basis of neurosis.

MASK A term coined by Stekel to refer to characterological artifice.

MASLOW, ABRAHAM (1908–1970). American psychologist who promoted the issue of a person's need system identified as a hierarchy of needs around which form various aspects of personality. The concept of actualization (approximating one's potential) gained its currency from Maslow.

MASOCHISM Named after the Austrian novelist Leopold von Sacher Masoch (1863–1895). Masochism refers to the person courting any number of painful situations, as if deriving covert pleasure from them. These can include sexual, aggressive, and humiliating circumstances. Freud originally speculated that masochism was sadism turned in toward the self. The more modern and general psychoanalytic position is that masochism represents a penance for underlying, unconscious guilt. This guilt is basically directed toward a historical nuclear family member, that is, a parent, and is reflexively repeated in the person's present life, as a playing out of repetition compulsion. Eventually, Freud developed a tripartite conception of masochism:

Feminine masochism—ostensible nature of passivity of the female.
Moral or ideal masochism—the need or desire for punishment to relieve guilt feelings evoked by a moral transgression such as persistent oedipal striving or fantasies.
Primary or erotogenic masochism—pain needed for sexual excitation and gratification.

MASOCHISTIC PERSONALITY DISORDER Equivalent to *Self-defeating personality disorder*. The masochistic person seeks punishment or pain, ostensibly to satisfy the need to assuage guilt. Psychoanalytically, this guilt may be underpinned by an impacted and historical unconscious anger (toward a parent) that generates a more conscious sense that "something is wrong." The something wrong can't be identified (because it is repressed), and this something is understood to be an underlying anger to which the guilt is related. Therefore, unless this repressed, unconsciously held anger is surfaced and understood, presumably the subject's masochistic inclination will endure. However, when the conflict is sublimated and the masochism not acted out, then, in a more positive sense (although still neurotic), we see individuals who are massively conscientious, true "workaholics." When they are at a point of working themselves to death, they can then breathe for a while because such tyrannical perseverance may have satisfied the requirement for a satisfaction of penance. However, because the underlying real conflict has not been identified and consequently worked out, the masochistic cycle starts to awaken and the quest for penance begins again—this being the pivotal engine for the emergence of the repetition-compulsion within the entire masochistic process as well. The underlying real conflict is the ostensible repressed anger toward a nuclear family member (a parent) that fuels the guilt igniting the entire process.

MASTERSON, JAMES F. (1926–). American psychiatrist/psychoanalyst. A pioneer contributor to self and object relations approaches to personality disorders and psychotherapy. A variety of contributions include investigations into abandonment, depression, and the borderline and narcissistic personalities. Founder and director of the Masterson Institute for Psychoanalytic Psychotherapy.

MASTURBATION Manipulation of sexual organs accompanied by sexual fantasies the purpose of which is to achieve sexual gratification either through orgasm or simply through the stimulation of erogenous zones. Compulsive masturbation is psychoanalytically considered an acting out because the inordinate attention to the masturbation and its habitual occurrence is ostensibly designed to avoid other more productive and even sublimating activities such as relating to another person. Psychologically, the acting out (like all acting out) is an attempt not to know something, and the compulsive masturbation thus keeps whatever needs to be known repressed and therefore unconscious.

MATERNAL DEPRIVATION SYNDROME Seen in children who, from an early time in their lives, are institutionalized or who have depriving mothers or depriving primary caregivers. Symptoms such as withdrawal as well as other depressive pathologies may be seen.

MATERNAL OVERPROTECTION Referring to any parental overmonitoring and control of the child, leading ultimately to passivity, dependence, suppressed anger, and the permanent immaturity that occurs in cases of arrested development.

MAY, ROLLO (1909–1994). American existential psychologist who was influenced by the American humanistic movement. He formulated what could be considered stages of development. These are

innocence—preself-conscious state of the infant, neither good nor bad;

rebellion—stage of childhood and adolescence, from the two year old's "no," to the adolescent's "no way": all in the service of ego development;

ordinary—normal adult ego, characterized by successful discharging of responsibilities;

creative—the authentic adult; this is the existential stage in which the person confronts the challenge of anxiety with courage.

Rollo May also formulated the interesting notion of the daimonic. This concept refers to the entire system of motives including what he calls the lower needs, such as food and sex, and the higher needs, such as love. A daimon is anything that obsesses a person—hence daimonic possession. This daimonic can become evil only if its balance is disrupted. The most important daimon is eros or love. May's concept of "will" correlates to the ability to organize oneself in the service of goal attainment. Implementing the will also relates to reality testing.

MDI Manic-depressive illness.

MEDIATING MECHANISMS A clinical reference to interstitial links between causal precipitators of an emotional/mental disorder and the disorder itself.

MEDIATION PROCESS See Cognitive mediation.

MEDICAL MINISTRY In Logotherapy, the medical ministry appeals to the healthy aspect of the individual in order to affect that person's attitude toward their own suffering. Especially targeted to individuals with resistive somatic complaints.

MEDICAL MODEL Referring to the results-oriented treatment of any disorder, not necessarily with regard to dynamic factors. Focus is on the target of treatment, and the focus on results awaits empirical confirmation.

MEGALOMANIA Defined as thoughts of greatness, omniscience, and omnipotence usually referred to as delusions of grandeur. According to Freud, energy of the libido, usually directed toward another, is rather self-endowed so that a narcissistic impulse is attributed to the subject. Synonym for grandiosity.

MELANCHOLIA Considered as a most severe depression with all attendant anhedonic symptoms; for example, loss of interest in pleasurable activities, loss of weight, and insomnia. See Depression.

MELANCHOLIA, HYPOCHONDRIACAL Depression with hypochondriasis usually considered within a schizophrenic personality. Complaints of stress are repetitive.

MELANCHOLIA, INVOLUTIONAL See Involutional psychosis.

MEMORY Other than a conventional definition of memory, a psychodynamic/psychoanalytic understanding of memory implies the importance of remembering historic data (in the sense of uncovering such memory) and strongly implicates repression, resistance, and transference as important constructs in the therapeutic endeavor.

MEMORY, EARLY Important in the psychodynamic understanding of character formation and the defense system. Ernest Schactel contributed to the literature on early amnesia and infancy.

MEMORY, SCREEN See Screen memory.

MEMORY, UNCONSCIOUS Memories of events and persons can presumably be relegated to the unconscious and thus available for access through a psychotherapeutic process. Bringing such memory to consciousness is thought to permit the accompanying affect to then be subject to analysis.

MEMORY TRACE Residue of a conscious realization that is not entirely repressed.

MENDACITY In clinical usage refers to pathological lying.

MENDICANCY, PATHOLOGICAL A person with this proclivity will plead and beg for money, even in the absence of need. A form of hoarding that reveals the tip of a more pathological underpinning.

MENNINGER, KARL AUGUSTUS (1893–1990). American psychiatrist who proposed the unitary theory of mental illness—an attempt to synthesize the organization of mental functioning. A member of the Menninger family—founders of the Menninger Clinic of Topeka, Kansas. Author of volumes *Man Against Himself* and *Love Against Hate*.

MENOPAUSE Gradual ending of menstruation in females, also called the involutional period. Symptoms may occur because of hormonal changes.

MENTALIZATION In developmental psychopathology and according to Fonagy and others, this refers to disordered relationships in the context of attachment theory; that is, the ability to understand one's mental state as well as the mental state of others requires decent development in the experience of attachment and relationship building. Therefore, when attachment is underachieved, mentalization suffers. Also applied in the context of neuropsychoanalytic thinking with respect to deficits of autism and schizophrenia. In addition, in this context, self-awareness is apparently seen as epigenetic; the essential function of the mind and brain is to organize experience in order to establish meaning. Mentalization means that the mind mediates experience and that such a process requires affect regulation that predates cognitive synthesis; with cognitive synthesis comes autobiographical memory.

MENTAL RETARDATION Conventionally considered of significantly below-average intelligence quotient.

MENTAL STATUS The psychiatric mental examination of a patient consisting of clinical impressions of the patient's appearance and behavior, and the patient's sensorium (comprised of memory, orientation, retention, abstraction ability, and judgment).

MERGER TRANSFERENCE See Transference.

MESMER, FRANZ ANTON (1773–1815). European physician noted as the first hypnotist. Hypnosis was then called Mesmerism. Magnets were first used with steel rods believed to facilitate the transfer of magnetic fluid designed to cure the patient.

MESOMORPH See Sheldon, William Herbert.

METAPHOR Seeking analogies in order to capture the essence of an idea. The representation of an idea with the substitution of some more figurative picture. Considered higher-order thinking unless constantly substituted for normal language, in which case such metaphoric thinking can resemble or be equivalent to basic primary process thinking, that is, the type of thinking that contains disjointedness in thought and registers raw emotion within the context of chaotic and dyscontrolled impulses.

METAPSYCHOLOGICAL PROFILE Anna Freud's contribution to the organization of clinical observations and overall data, correlating psychological / emotional symptoms to the person's repressed unconscious material.

METAPSYCHOLOGY Freud's term for theoretical abstraction.

METHADONE A substitute agent in the treatment of heroin addiction. Although also creating dependence, the drug is nevertheless helpful because of the absence of typical heroin addictive effects, such as the need for ever higher dosages.

METONYMY In some cases of schizophrenia, a person will use words or phrases that are not at all precise yet are related to the word or phrase that was meant. Hypothesized to reflect abnormal interaction during critical phases of development.

MICROCOSM OF WORDS See Words, microcosm of.

MICROPSYCHOSIS See Pseudoneurotic schizophrenia.

MIGRAINE Severe headache (but also significantly and qualitatively different from a bad headache) with accompanying symptoms such as nausea, visual auras, and photophobia (painful light sensitivity). Treated by many psychotherapists as a phenomenon caused by stress and intense conflict.

MIGRAINE, NEURALGIA A cluster migraine characterized by excruciating pulsating pain.

MILLON, THEODORE (1928–). European born American psychologist. Known as the grandfather of personality theory. Contribution to personality theory includes his theory of the role of personality in an integrated conception of psychopathology. His is also an evolutionary model of personality. His personality test, The Millon Clinical Multiaxial Inventory is one of the most utilized of personality tests. See Millon Clinical Multiaxial Inventory.

MILLON CLINICAL MULTIAXIAL INVENTORY (MCMI). A true / false personality index that measures twenty-four scales composed of four groups: clinical personality patterns, severe personality pathology, clinical syndromes, and severe clinical syndromes. Developed by Theodore Millon.

MIND In psychoanalysis, mind is more or less equivalent to psyche or the psychic apparatus. See Neuropsychoanalysis.

MINDFULNESS Becoming aware of what you have previously done on automatic pilot by simply observing your emotions without getting caught up in them.

MINDFULNESS MEDITATION Technique increasingly used in cognitive behavior therapy. Involves training in breathing and relaxation accompanied by observing emotional reactions and the accompanying thoughts in a detached way, without trying to control or pass judgment on them, until a state of calm is achieved.

MINUCHIN, SALVADOR (1921–). Argentinian physician. Family theorist / therapist who developed family therapy known as structured family therapy (SFT). SFT yields diagrammatic family parameters. It is a systems-oriented therapy that focuses on interactions or transactions within the subsystems of the family. Some concepts utilized to understand the infrastructural mechanisms of the family include enmeshment, permeability, coalitions, restructuring, and unbalancing. Objective is to unstructure and then restructure the family. See Family therapy.

MIRRORING See Selfobject functions.

MIRROR SIGN A phenomenon seen with schizophrenic patients who can find themselves staring into a mirror for undue amounts of time and, occasionally, grimacing as well. Generally interpreted as reflecting a sense of doubt with respect to the self: "Am I who I am?" In the normal sense, seen also with adolescents as an indication of such doubt. Can also mean the inability to recognize oneself as reflecting a brain anomaly or a deeper psychopathological symptom.

MISANTHROPY A characterological paranoialike attitude reflecting distrust of individuals specifically and the hating of mankind generally.

MISIDENTIFICATION Two types of the misidentification are

Amnesic type—confusion of consciousness.

Delusional type—inability to recognize the object because of the belief that the object has already been transformed by some outside force.

MISOGAMY Particular aversion to marriage.

MISOGYNY Hatred of women.

MITCHELL, STEPHEN A. (1943–2001). American psychologist/psychoanalyst who, along with Jay Greenberg, ushered in the synthesis they referred to as relational interpersonal theory. Mitchell was instrumental in moving the field of psychoanalysis toward a relational perspective and away from psychoanalytic drive theory. See Relational psychotherapy.

MMPI (MINNESOTA MULTIPHASIC PERSONALITY INVENTORY) A personality test designed to assess diagnosis and personality type. Ten scales are designed to measure

Hypochondriasis—concern with bodily functions.
Depression—poor morale.
Hysteria—trigger level of stress.
Psychopathic—social deviation.
Masculinity-femininity—identification with one's gender role.
Paranoia—ideas of reference.
Psychasthenia—obsessive-compulsive, guilt.
Schizophrenia—bizarre thought.
Mania—elevated mood.
Social introversion—withdrawal.

MNEMIC Essentially meaning memory trace, as in a mnemic image.

MODALITY, THERAPEUTIC Any distinctive type of therapy treatment, usually consisting of a particular theoretical underpinning.

MODALITY PROFILE In multimodal behavior therapy, this profile consists of a list of treatments for the patient's corresponding problems.

MODELING In behavior therapy, this is learning through imitation.

MODEL SCENES Salient recollections of events in the patient's life that throw light on some aspect of the patient's current life. Developed by Lichtenberg, and elaborated by Lichtenberg and Lachmann to indicate the patient's organization of experience as it emerges in the current analysis. These scenes are cocreated by the patient and analyst to describe a pattern derived from what had been known.

MODELL, ARNOLD H. (1926–). American psychiatrist/psychoanalyst who within the confines of object relations theory investigated the conflict between a person's need for dependence and a corresponding need for autonomy. Also considered self psychology as an object relations theory. Modell investigated the correspondence of psychoanalytic precepts to those of neuroscience.

MOMENT OF MEETING This concept refers to the condition in which intersubjective relational knowing leads to a high-level affective experience between therapist and patient. It is an accurate sensing that permits a mutational event to occur, which enables a quantum shift in the therapy—equivalent to a new synthesis.

MONGOLISM Archaic term for Down's syndrome.

MONOMANIA An encapsulated psychosis during which other aspects of the person's functioning seem reasonably normal.

MOOD In a clinical sense usually refers to the range of overall emotional disposition from gloomy to elated or with respect to the sense of a swing of mood from one emotional disposition to its opposite. In psychoanalytic understanding, these poles are usually considered elation and depression or optimism and pessimism. In contrast to emotion considered to be transitory, mood is seen as containing a sustained presence.

MOOD DISORDERS Synonymous with affective disorders.

MORALITY, SPHINCTER In the psychology of Sandor Ferenczi, this concept refers to toilet training and its relation to the parents' dos and don'ts that are incorporated (or introjected) by the child and, in addition, presage the development of superego.

MORAL MASOCHISM See Masochism.

MORENO, J. L. (1892–1974). European-born American physician who introduced the modality referred to as psychodrama, essentially one Moreno created from his work in utilizing sociometrical analyses of how people behaved and interacted in groups. He then developed role-playing techniques among a host of other approaches in the uncovering of a person's feelings and motives and was essentially antipsychoanalytic insofar as he felt that psychodramatic involvement was a more direct and efficacious approach to the goals of therapy.

MORES, SOCIAL Major societal values that guide a person's behavior in contrast to folkways that are also included in the person's moral makeup, but in a minor key.

MORITA THERAPY Conceived by psychiatrist Shoma Morita of Japan (1874–1938). A form of reality therapy (phenomenological reality) including actual work experience, encouragement, and even so-called hard love, all of which is embodied in a communal setting. Said to be effective especially with hypochondriacal patients. It is a therapy that stresses the cultivation of character while focusing less on symptoms.

MORON A pejorative term for individuals who test significantly lower than average on IQ tests. Equivalent to retarded.

MORPHOLOGY The science of the structure of systems.

MORTIDO Federn's concept equivalent to Freud's destrudo, the destructive instinct.

MOTHER, COMPLETE A concept by Federn that is relegated to the fantasy life of schizophrenics, who presumably had mothers who were ambivalent about their role as mother and in their ambivalence demonstrated resentment and regret about the role. The schizophrenic, it is thought, then ruminates the idealized complete mother who in the fantasy accepts her role in a positive pure state so that the schizophrenic person feels finally satisfied in the acquisition of mother love.

MOTHER, GOOD ENOUGH See Winnicott, D. W.

MOTHER, PHALLIC Freud's notion of the male child's early fantasy that the mother possesses a penis based on the child's increasing awareness of his own penis. Through a series of developmental phases, rather than become obsessed with this idea, the child presumably then imposes a reaction formation to this idea that in turn produces feelings of disgust rather than attraction. How this is worked out figures rather prominently in various psychic developmental implications in the child's personality. In more conventional psychoanalytic terms, the phallic mother is usually seen as the assertive and aggressive mother.

MOTHER, SCHIZOPHRENOGENIC See Schizophrenogenic mother.

MOTILITY DISORDER A disorder of motion or gestures usually ascribed to catatonic patients.

MOTIVATION Its clinical relevance is basically tied to the concepts of immediate needs for gratification versus the postponement of gratification in the service of longer-range goals. The latter state implies greater maturity, while the former state implies more immaturity.

MOTIVATION, UNCONSCIOUS The pursuit of goals involving patterns of behavior that correspond to these goals, although such motivation is not consciously crystallized.

MOTOR SKILLS DISORDER Referring essentially to difficulty in coordination.

MOURNING The grief experience to loss, presumably resulting in the relinquishment of the object. A sample of theoreticians who have contributed to the literature in the psychology of mourning include Freud, Fairbairn, Kavaler-Adler, and Masterson.

MULTIAXIAL CLASSIFICATION In the psychiatric (*DSM*) nomenclature, the multiaxial classification consists of several constituent dimensions on which to assess a patient's diagnosis and prognosis. The major diagnostic entities of this multiaxial classification system are included on Axis I and Axis II. See Axis I and II.

MULTIMODAL THERAPY The psychological approach to treatment should consist of a targeting of each facet of the person's existence. The enumeration of these facets of the person's experience is based upon the Basic ID, an aspect of behavior therapy developed by Arnold Lazarus. See Basic ID.

MULTIPLE PERSONALITY DISORDER (MPD) See Dissociative disorders.

MUNCHHAUSEN SYNDROME Named for the fictitious Baron Munchhausen, who exaggerated tales of illness. Such persons are called hospital hoboes, because they seek hospitalization at any given opportunity. They will feign illness even to the extent of undergoing surgery. In children, it is suspected that the mother (or primary caregiver) manipulates the issue so that the child begins to demonstrate symptoms of whatever disease is discussed. It has also been attributed to psychopathic malingering in adults. As a psychodynamic consideration, secondary gain for attention is frequently considered in the etiology of this syndrome.

MURRAY, HENRY A. (1893–1988). Influential American psychologist who developed the Thematic Apperception Test (TAT)—a projective testing approach that invites subjects to tell a story involving past, present, and future events in the presentation of an ambiguous scene. The stories that are created reveal underlying attitudes, emotions, and motivations as well as a host of other considerations of the subject's personality. For the greater part of the twentieth century, the TAT, along with the Rorschach Test and the Machover Draw a Person Test, comprised the basic standard projective battery applied in psychological testing.

MUTATIVE INTERPRETATION As a result of therapeutic interpretation, this refers to a salient or signal shift in the patient's set personality organization. As a function of the patient's understanding, a sudden sense of a difference in internal experience is achieved. This is an important therapeutic concept insofar as it represents a benchmark in the therapeutic endeavor. Also referred to as mutative therapeutic moment.

MUTISM A condition of silence whereby the person does not easily utter any kind of verbal communicative message. However, there are variations of mutism. One such variation is not named but can be called hypomutism (somewhat less severe than mutism). In hypomutism, the person may not be able to initiate conversation (existing within the context of an unstructured situation—that is to say, a social situation), and yet such a person will always be able to answer direct questions (even within the social situation). Within a structured situation such as a workplace, the mutism may be entirely nullified, and the person can indeed initiate or implement verbal communication in the service of the job.

MUTISM, ELECTIVE Usually seen in children. With a change of venue or environment, the withdrawal of verbal communication can cease. Also referred to as selective mustism.

MYASTHENIA Muscle weakness frequently attributed to depression. Also sometimes seen in schizophrenic patients.

MYOCLONIC SLEEP Characterized by knee jerks during sleep and seen frequently with people who suffer from insomnia.

N

NAIKAN THERAPY A treatment associated with Morita therapy utilizing the patient's own guilt as a motivating force. The sense of obligation and community responsibility constitutes an underpinning to the treatment and is said to be curative with criminals. In Japanese, *naikan* means looking inward, as in self-reflection.

NAIL-BITING Usually a chronic symptom understood psychoanalytically as an expression of tension concerned with the experience of thwarted needs and ambition. Associated with the sense of frustration and inexorable impatience. Also related to derivative anal conflict, ultimately having obsessional implications. May reflect an attempt to control anger insofar as nails can symbolize weapons.

NAKHLA, FAYEK (1933–). Egyptian-born American psychiatrist. Has published on the therapeutic process and is an exponent of object relations. Member, British Psychoanalytic Society and editorial board, *Dictionary of Psychopathology.*

NARCISSISM Usually defined as self-love and self-interest with a distinct absence of empathy. Omniscience, omnipotence, and grandiosity are characteristics of the personality. The false sense of self with respect to omnipotent feelings is termed *primary narcissism.* Of course, reality interferes, and the narcissist's wishes then become frequently thwarted. This is probably the best definition of a reality check. A so-called secondary narcissism can then develop in which the superego (the sense of right and wrong) begins to love the ego; under such conditions, the narcissistic person begins to feel that, although wishes are not automatically granted, they are felt to be justified in the first place. In the narcissist, sexuality is always in the service of the person's grandiosity. In Freudian theory, the theoretical makeup of narcissism concerns how the id generates the libidinous energy that services the ego. Classically considered a sexual perversion in which the subject's body constitutes the narcissistic focus. The person uses denial, displacement, and grandiose justification for expressing needs, rather than acknowledging some other obvious physical or personality problem. Synonymous with egocentric. A distinction also needs to be cited between normal (healthy) narcissism and pathological narcissism. Further, narcissistic rage is a reaction to narcissistic injury, and this reflects a breakdown in self-cohesion. Contributors to the literature on narcissism include Akhtar, Cooper, H. Deutsch, Fiscalini, Giovacchini, Kernberg, Kohut, Masterson, Morrison, Ornstein, Rothstein.

NARCISSISTIC NEUROSIS A particular narcissistic pathology whereby the subject, who may be a patient in psychotherapy, is frequently unable to form a transference largely because, according to Freud, libido is absorbed by the ego and not directed toward external instinctual objects. Narcissistic neurosis contrasts with transference neurosis. See Transference neurosis.

NARCISSISTIC PERSONALITY DISORDER Essentially, the meaning of a personality disorder as understood clinically and diagnostically, refers to the person's absence of concern or anxiety regarding fixed patterns of relating and behavior. Thus the behavior is considered to be ego-syntonic (the person is not bothered by it). The

DSM narcissistic personality is one such personality disorder consisting of an overfocus on self-interest, an exaggerated grandiosity, lack of empathy, inappropriate sense of entitlement, and relentless search for ego gratification, usually in the form of needing to be aggrandized and adored. See Personality / character disorder.

NARCISSISTIC RAGE Related to a rage reaction to the experience of humiliation. In large part more typically seen in men. See Narcissism.

NARCISSISTIC SUPPLIES Anything that nourishes and contributes to the patient's self-esteem, including flattery or adoration.

NARCISSISTIC WOUND Criticism toward the subject that injures or wounds self-esteem.

NARCOLEPSY Excessive Daytime Sleepiness (EDS). In *DSM* nosology considered to be a dyssomnia. Narcolepsy is inherited and may also be seen in animals. It can be reasonably controlled with medication. The narcoleptic syndrome or tetrad of symptoms is comprised of

narcolepsy itself—the compelling need to sleep;

cataplexy—the loss of voluntary musculature to the stimulus of intense emotion (usually sudden, with an emphasis on the emotion of surprise);

sleep paralysis—a sense of paralysis either upon entering sleep or upon awakening;

hypnagogic hallucination—in which the subject (usually during the sleep paralysis) has a dream that is experienced as so real that, upon awakening, the person is never sure as to whether it was actually a dream or actually happened.

NARCOTIC Sleep-inducing drug that generates a feeling of well-being. It is addictive and also induces sleep.

NATIONAL PSYCHOLOGICAL ASSOCIATION FOR PSYCHOANALYSIS See Reik, Theodor.

NECROMANCY The belief that a person can predict future events by communicating with dead spirits.

NECROPHILIA A paraphilia (perversion). In this case, the perverse impulse is sexual and directed by the wish to connect with the love object—a dead person—in order to achieve orgasm. Implies the wish to avoid any kind of sexual interfacing that could be considered an interpersonal challenge so that the acting out of this particular perversion is, for the subject, an empowerment: no one talks back.

NEED Clinically, need is seen as related to the pleasure principle, wishes, and instinct. It is also intricately connected to feelings of deprivation, anger, and the birth of symptoms, especially when the essence of the need is thwarted.

Need-fear dilemma—applied to schizophrenic individuals who become more comfortable in a structured setting such as a hospital, but, at the same time, feel apprehensive and worried about authoritarian control.

Need, neurotic—Karen Horney's concept that the person needs to be considered by others in the way in which the subject wishes, such as, for example, with respect and admiration.

NEED-SATISFYING OBJECT Any object (person) that loves and aims to satisfy the subject. Mainly referring to the infant's attachment to mother or the primary care giver, who automatically satisfies the infant's needs.

NEGATION Any untoward experience is, in part, softened by focusing on its positive corollary. For example, it's not that the subject failed the test. Rather, it's that the subject thinks about its fortune to have not failed other tests.

NEGATIVE AUTOMATIC THOUGHTS (NATS) In cognitive behavior therapy, these are thoughts below the level of consciousness. In Beck's cognitive theory of depression, cognitive symptoms of depression precede depressive mood, therefore negative thoughts are seen to be key elements in the appearance of depression. See Automatic thoughts.

NEGATIVE OEDIPUS COMPLEX Subject chooses same-gender parent to love and considers the opposite-gender parent as a rival.

NEGATIVE PERIOD, FIRST In very young children, negative responses become a normal phase of the developmental process—to wit, the terrible twos.

NEGATIVE PERSONALITY DISORDER See Passive-aggressive personality.

NEGATIVE PRACTICE See Paradoxical therapy.

NEGATIVE REINFORCEMENT See Reinforcement.

NEGATIVE THERAPEUTIC REACTION This is equivalent to the psychoanalytic concept of resistance in treatment and is ascribed to superego rigidity. The negative therapeutic reaction is usually seen with patients who are severely masochistic. It is also seen with obsessional patients, borderline, and paranoid types.

NEGATIVE TRANSFERENCE See Transference resistance.

NEGATIVE TRIAD In Beck's cognitive theory of depression, a person who is depressed has an overly negative and pessimistic view of the self, others, and the future. This triad is connected to certain cognitive distortions such as selective abstraction, all-or-nothing thinking, and overgeneralization, processes that significantly influence the person's mood, sense of worth, and ability to reach his or her goals. See Cognitive distortions.

NEGATIVISM Usually seen as protest behavior and may be ascribed to the person's need for power. It can also take the form of a passive-aggressive approach in which the aim of the protest is to render the object helpless—to reduce the power of the other and, by implication, to enhance the power of the self. Psychoanalytically, it can be seen also as an attempt to increase the impermeability of one's boundary, and is frequently the psychological culprit in the avoidance of commitment to any possible primary relationship.

NEO-FREUDIANISM Those psychoanalysts who proceed in their therapeutic encounters using a good part of Freudian theory, while incorporating their own theoretical formulations that actually modify certain Freudian precepts and then correspondingly appear in neo-Freudian form in the treatment. Examples include the work of Adler, Horney, Fromm, and Sullivan. In most cases, the neo- Freudians become more interpersonal in the treatment so that the "blank screen" of classical Freudian psychoanalysis is the basic apparent modification of the neo-Freudians, with a tendency to move away from instinct theory. Many therapies based upon relational theories are included.

NEOLOGISM Condensations of words and phrases peculiar to the particular individual, spoken without intention to condense or to confuse. These are occasionally quite interesting, but in repetitive or extreme form are products of schizophrenic thinking. This sort of schizophrenic product is considered syncretistic (correlational) thinking in which associational links of words yield a phrase that seems nonsensical but, if traced to its origin, will reveal a serial linkage of synonyms and associative connections that do, in fact, reveal its sense.

NEOPHASIA, POLYGLOT Synthetic language created by an individual that is entirely idiosyncratic.

NETWORK THERAPY A therapy program popular in the 1960s identifying and creating an environment around the patient that comprises nuclear family members as well as an entire population—a universe of the patient's life—including friends, relatives, and other interested relevant individuals. For this kind of therapy, a large room is selected that can accommodate scores of people. Therapist assistants roam this so-called universe and begin to uncover secrets. At some point, an important secret is "blown," and results have been reported that claim miraculous shifts in pathology. Some have reported one hundred or more people in the network session.

NEURASTHENIA Referring to easy fatigability and physical weakness. As a psychological symptom, it is considered akin to a hypochondriacal defensive posture, and individuals who display this symptom are thought to be repressing anger. This diagnostic phenomenon was frequently reported in the late nineteenth and early twentieth centuries, and in the first *Diagnostic and Statistical Nomenclature* of the American Psychiatric Association, published in 1952, was referred to as a psychophysiologic reaction. It has been hypothesized by some as related to a new presumed functional state referred to as chronic fatigue syndrome.

NEUROPSYCHOANALYSIS A branch of neuropsychology, the interface between psychoanalysis and neuroscience. Essentially, it is an attempt to make more visible the relation of mind to brain. It is the science that deals with the relationship between behavior and the mind, on the one hand, and the nervous system, especially the brain, on the other. In light of the definition of psychoanalysis as the scientific study of the unconscious mind, the discipline of neuropsychoanalysis studies the relationship between the functions of the unconscious mind and the brain systems that process information at a nonconscious level.

The hard problem—In the field of neuropsychoanalysis, bridging the difference between mind and brain is considered the hard problem.

Dual aspect monism—Also referred to as perspectivism. It is the attempt to understand the so-called hard problem, that is, that brain and mind are monastic (composed of the same cells), although perceived by the self in two different ways. The brain is understood objectively (as through surgery), while the mind can be understood through insight, introspection, and various kinds of paper and pencil tests.

Luminaries in this relatively new domain of neuroscience include Antonio Damasio, Aikaterini Fotopoulou, Eric Kandel, Joseph LeDoux, Helen Mayberg, Jaak Panksepp, Allan Schore, Howard Shevrin, Karen Kaplan-Solms, Oliver H. Turnbull, and Yoram Yovell. Mark Solms is credited as the founder of the field.

NEUROPSYCHOANALYSIS OF OEDIPAL BEHAVIOR According to Fisher, and in the domain of neuropsychoanalysis, lust can be correlated to a testosterone-driven system, romantic love to a dopamine-driven system, and attachment behavior to an oxytocin-driven system.

NEUROPSYCHOLOGY A psychological specialty in which psychologists assess for brain damage, brain dysfunction, and level of impairment, utilizing a variety of paper and pencil tests as well as clinical diagnostic observation. See Neuropsychoanalysis.

NEUROSIS The psychoneuroses were traditionally differentiated from the psychoses and from the character or personality disorders. The neuroses were seen to be characterized by the presence of felt or experienced anxiety, but not poor reality testing (which is the case in psychosis). Character or personality disorders were those patterns of behavior, traits of personality, or patterns of functioning that were not accompanied by any tension or anxiety, despite the fact that, in many cases, such behavior would result in self-defeating ends. Thus, in the neuroses, the anxiety signal can be valuable in treatment because such anxiety alerts the individual to whatever may be the deleterious consequences of problematic behavior, acting as a motivator for treatment. Examples of neuroses include anxiety neurosis, obsessional and compulsive neurosis, and hysterical neurosis.

Neurosis, anxiety—See anxiety neurosis.

Neurosis, iatrogenic—See Iatrogeny.

Neurosis, malignant—the exaggeration of a neurotic symptom that begins to disable the person. An example would be an agoraphobia that develops out of a mild social anxiety ultimately leading to the condition in which the person may not be able to leave the bedroom—or even the bed. Of course, in such cases, the malignancy of the neurosis is such that a psychoticlike rigidity develops, and then prevails.

Neurosis, mixed—in the diagnostic nomenclature, a mixed neurosis consists of a diagnosis that contains components of various diagnoses. For example, a diagnosis could be obsessive-compulsive with passive-aggressive and depressive features.

Neurosis, obsessional—See Obsessive-compulsive psychoneurosis.

Neurosis, performance—equivalent to performance anxiety typically seen with stage performers.

Neurosis, transference—See Transference neurosis.

Neurosis, traumatic—disturbed behavior or feeling as a function of a trauma, then translated into psychological symptomatology.

NEUROTICISM Rather than responding in a more objective manner to external stimuli, neuroticism reflects a contamination by the person's strong internal signal interposed on perception of the outside world, thereby inviting a particular idiosyncratic response. This idiosyncrasy is represented by the person's so-called negative feelings such as anxiety, shame, shyness, self-consciousness, depression, or anger. Such individuals are not terribly resilient and therefore exaggerate potential threat from the outside world as well as experiencing frustration in an exaggerated way.

NEUROTIC NEED A Horneyan concept. See Need.

NEUROTIC RESIGNATION See Resignation, neurotic.

NEW YORK PSYCHOANALYTIC INSTITUTE See Brenner, Charles.

NGRI An acronym meaning "not guilty by reason of insanity."

NIGHT EATING Seen in obese patients and associated with symptoms of next-day anorexia and insomnia. Psychologically seen as a function of anxiety, anger, a sense of failure, helplessness, and even underachievement.

NIGHTMARE Typically defined as a dream that frightens and therefore awakens the dreamer. However, according to Kellerman, any dream in which the content of the dream awakens the dreamer should be considered a nightmare. The salient criterion of the nightmare, therefore, is that the content of the dream can create an awakening with a number of affects—other than fear—that can satisfy this criterion. Such awakenings can occur in scenarios of the dream in which, for example, the dreamer awakens to the emotion of

acceptance—the moment of the dream in which a sense of complete idealized contentment is experienced;

anticipation—the moment of the dream in which intense expectation or anticipation is experienced as something urgent;

anger at and/or aggression—a situation in which the dreamer becomes furious or rageful and attacks some figure in the dream;

disgust—situation whereby the dreamer becomes nauseated and awakens in a mood of revulsion;

ecstasy—in which the dreamer awakens because of a sexual overstimulation resulting in orgasm or almost in orgasm;

fear—the moment of the dream in which intense fear or terror is experienced;

sorrow—a scene where a figure dies and the dreamer begins to sob and then awakens;

surprise—the punch line of a joke, usually that the dreamer hears told by someone else.

Thus, obviously, awakening to fear is not the only content of the dream that can identify or define the dream as a nightmare or cause it to become a nightmare. Presumably, the nightmare is more likely to occur if the dreamwork mechanisms of displacement, symbolization, condensation, and secondary elaboration weaken so that the barrier is lowered against the appearance of primary process material—and this includes activation of intense emotional responses.

NIGHT RESIDUE See Residue, night.

NIGHT TERROR A sleep phenomenon in children usually up until puberty. Equivalent to an intense nightmare in the absence of REM (Rapid Eye Movement) or even with no memory of a dream. The child awakens in terror and may become exceedingly disturbed—even to the extent of fleeing.

NIHILISTIC DELUSION Considered an existential delusion that raises the question Do we exist or not? In this delusion the answer is a resounding "not."

NOCTURNAL EMISSION Orgasmic emission of seminal fluid, usually during sleep, in the absence of actual interpersonal sexual contact.

NOCTURNAL MYOCLONUS Jerking of the leg muscles during sleep in the absence of painful or uncomfortable sensations. Part of the diagnosis Disorders of Initiating and Maintaining Sleep (DIMS) or, in the *DSM* nomenclature, known as part of the dyssomnias, including insomnia.

NOMADISM Highly unusual phenomenon related to a person's tendency to wander and drift from place to place. Can be a result of both organic or psychogenic factors.

NOMENCLATURE Essentially meaning nosology or the classification of disorders.

NOMOLOGICAL NETWORK Any system of correlational variables regarding a focal point embraced by a theoretical matrix. Therefore a nomological network is essentially synonymous with the phrase *theoretical network* or with the idea of the internal consistency of a theoretical network.

NON COMPOS MENTIS Unknowing and not responsible for one's actions because of mental impairment.

NONDIRECTIVE PSYCHOTHERAPY See Rogers, Carl.

NOOGENIC NEUROSIS In logotherapy, an existential vacuum leading to the formation of symptoms. Relates to the experience of frustration.

NOSOLOGY See Nomenclature.

NOT-ME Harry Stack Sullivan's concept of the denial of personal experience when the trauma is too much to manage. The person then disassociates from the experience and refuses to accept it as having actually happened. Through the mechanism of repression, the event is then presumably held in the unconscious until the trauma, through the probing of some stimulus, is brought to quasi consciousness, which elicits the response of "It's not-me." This is different from the simple denial that accompanies conscious realization of a traumatic event, in which the sufferer refuses to yield to the so-called facts. Sullivan goes on to describe what he terms "uncanny emotions" surrounding such traumatic memories. These uncanny emotions are dread, terror, and even loathing.

NREM (Non Rapid Eye Movement). The four stages of sleep without dreams.

NUCLEAR CONFLICT The person's central problem.

NUCLEAR FAMILY One's original family.

NYMPHOMANIA Female hypersexuality.

O

OBEDIENCE, AUTOMATIC Complete obedience on the part of the person in the absence of any critical or independent thinking. Sometimes seen in catatonic or exceedingly dependent patients.

OBEDIENCE, DEFERRED Freud's notion that any command by an authority figure, early in one's life, can be resisted at first, but some stimulus later on can call forth the need to comply. This idea contains profound implications for the psychology of transference as well as illuminating motives and behavior of larger social-psychological phenomena.

OBESITY Excessive body weight of more than 20 percent of what is considered normal.

OBJECT Originally defined by Freud as the tropistic direction of the instinct by which the instinct achieves its aim or goal. The "object of the instinct," is the manner in which the relation of instinct to object is described. In modern psychoanalytic terminology or in clinical object-relations theory, the object generally refers to another person, as in the relationship of subject to object.

OBJECT, INTERNAL An internal object is an integral part of the person's psychic structure formed from the early significant caretaking relationship. Later external object relations can modify this internal structure. Introjection puts the external object inside, so that it becomes an internal object representation or a dynamic and visceral object that is protosymbolic. The introjections are presumed to be played out in fantasy.

OBJECT CATHEXIS Referring to the emotional or psychic energy invested in another person, external object.

OBJECT CHOICE Usually a euphemism for object love—the one invested with love, who can also be a self-representation (narcissistic).

OBJECT CONSTANCY The ability to sustain a mature relationship. This is considered difficult because relationships need to be worked on and, along with being potentially nourishing, are also frequently stress producing. Retaining object constancy challenges the ego and therefore requires good, or at least reasonable, ego strength to withstand the pressures and stresses of working on the relationship. In object relations theory, a successful traversing of the separation-individuation process will lead to the ability to sustain object constancy. As a function of the child's experience of others (and also as related to self), during approximately the first three years, perception of the world (to the extent that it is either loving or hostile) determines such inner constancy. It is the anchoring of the child's inner life as it becomes consolidated and, to whatever extent, adaptive.

OBJECT INCONSTANCY Frequently seen in borderline personalities, where sustaining the relationship is almost impossible because of the subject's inability to tolerate relationship frustration—a frustration that in turn usually generates eruptive behavior.

OBJECT LIBIDO Libido (mental or sexual energy) invested in others (in objects). Refers to another person, about whom the subject is interested, in contrast to narcissistic libido where the subject is invested in the self.

OBJECT LOSS The loss of the external object leading to mourning.

OBJECT LOVE The person (other than the self) that is loved.

OBJECT RELATIONS THEORY A theory of development based upon the organization of relationships, in contrast to a Freudian approach that is based upon the alleviation of instinctual tension. Object relations theory is essentially a paradigm for understanding how the external world is internalized. It is a model that explains mental functioning, both intrapsychic and interpersonal, on the basis of internalized elements of personality and psychic structures. The British school focuses on the significance of the infant-mother experience. Some proponents of object relations theory include Balint, Bion, Bollas, Bowlby, Fairbairn, Guntrip, Hoffman, Kavaler-Adler, Kernberg, Klein, M., Kohut, Kosseff, Mahler, Masterson, Mitchell, Racker, Seinfeld, Slochower, Spitz, Stern, Suttie, and Winnicott.

OBJECT RELATIONSHIP Relation of subject and object; that is, the mutual reciprocal interaction with external objects and the person's established intrapsychic personality structure. Person to other.

OBJECT REPRESENTATION The mental representation of an object. It is different from an internal object, which is part of the self structure.

OBJECT USAGE See Winnicott, D. W.

OBSESSION A repetitive focus on an idea, person, or circumstance that is almost entirely resistant to conscious control. As a symptom (and presumably, like all symptoms), it represents a repression of anger toward a specific person (also repressed) and, as such, this obsessive rumination reflects the thwarting of a wish. It is assumed that the specific person toward whom the subject is angry is the one who thwarted the wish. Intrusive thoughts are products of obsessive rumination. See Symptom.

OBSESSIONAL CHARACTER A person who has translated obsessional proclivities into patterns of behavior as well as attitudes. Thus, such individuals display controlling needs and behaviors, tidiness, overconscientiousness, as well as a focus on intellectual and rational approaches to relationships. The character traits of this type are all designed to keep anxiety at a distance.

OBSESSIONAL DEFENSE SYSTEM Obsessional defenses are those that ostensibly keep aggressive and sexual impulses in check and the ego therefore remains safe from the invasion of instinctual forces. These defenses include reaction formation (turning attraction into disgust), isolation (separating emotion from ideas), and undoing (keeping new stimuli that could tempt the person from entering and/or remaining in the psyche). In addition, intellectualization and rationalization are other defenses utilized to aid in sustaining the need for control, as is the search or yearning for symmetry.

OBSESSIONAL THINKING Such a person utilizes intellectualization, rationalization, and logic to manage all the ambivalences that are relentlessly generated in all relationships. Although not due to any democratic leanings, such persons use conditional phrases and are always straining to see both sides of the issue. Abstraction, obliqueness, and indirection are typical because of the person's need for control.

OBSESSIVE-COMPULSIVE The modern *DSM* nomenclature refers to obsessive-compulsive reactions in two ways:

- *Obsessive-compulsive disorder*—This is considered to be an Axis I anxiety disorder insofar as such a person is prone to ruminating on one issue and then feeling the compelling need to follow through in behavior. An example will be the person who ruminates about locking the door at night and then generates doubt as to whether it was actually done so that the compelling need is to repeatedly check the locks. The rumination is the obsession, and the checking of the locks is the compulsion—thinking and doing—forming a ritual. Repetitive thoughts or even intrusive thoughts are causes of anxiety, and although such a person tries to become distracted from these experiences the obsessive preoccupation always prevails. Compulsions include hand washing and counting fantasies as well as other numerous ritualistic behaviors about which the subject is aware, while helpless to change. As a neurosis, the symptom will generate anxiety in the subject.
- *Obsessive-compulsive personality disorder*—This is considered to be an Axis II personality disorder in which orderliness, accountability to rules and regulations, perfectionistic needs, overconscientiousness, adherence to strict standards, extreme single-mindedness, hoarding, and general rigidity are characteristics of the personality. This obsessive-compulsive system requires a number of defense mechanisms that are brought to bear on the threat of impulses gaining the ascendancy, so that the idea of the return of the repressed gains currency here insofar as a fear of any loss of control becomes a first order of business. Thus, psychoanalytically, the psychodynamics of this process concerns the need to control impulse and, further, also implies that such underlying impulse is strong and

persistent. In psychoanalytic terms the impulse will be identified either as aggressive or sexual. See Repressed, return of the.

OBSTIPATION Severe constipation in children occasioned also by soiling. This is a symptom associated with suppressed anger. In treatment, the therapist is always interested in identifying the object (parent, close relative, or friend), with whom the child is frustrated and angry. It is usually the case that the culprit in this drama makes the child feel helpless and at a loss to know what to do about it.

OCCUPATIONAL NEUROSIS A symptom that directly affects the person's performance on the job. Stage actors may experience extreme stage fright to the extent that the actor may postpone performing or may even feign illness. In professional sports, certain athletes may lose proficiency—to wit, being unable to throw accurately. As in all symptoms, such occupational neurosis is reputed to reflect repressed anger toward a specific object that the subject targets as the responsible culprit in thwarting some important wish. See Symptom.

OCCUPATIONAL THERAPY Helping patients with concrete work production and / or activities of daily living in order to promote motivation and self-esteem.

OCEANIC FEELING The sense of being at one with the universe. Can be seen as reflecting omnipotent feelings or even megalomania, and is associated also with delusions of grandeur. See Archaic ego state; Omnipotence.

OEDIPAL Referring to the Oedipus complex and implying that the person's problem is related to some competitive striving concerning another same-gender person in relation to that person's significant other. Psychoanalytically, it is essentially a derivative of the wish to conquer or possess the parent of the opposite sex, displacing the rival. Thus clinical psychodynamic reference to something oedipal includes issues of competitiveness, possessiveness, and sexuality that conventionally involve two individuals of the same sex and one of the opposite sex—the oedipal triangle. See Neuropsychoanalysis of oedipal behavior.

OEDIPUS COMPLEX Introduced by Freud as a core, universal aspect of development and the key basis for the genesis of neurosis. It involves the triangular relationship that develops between the child and the same-sex and opposite-sex parent. Freud took the name from a Greek myth elaborated in Sophocles' drama in which a royal couple's son, Oedipus, is prophesied at birth to be fated to kill his father and marry his mother. In contemporary terms, the inevitability of character or personality to dictate decisions takes the place of fate. Freud proposed that a parallel psychological drama unfolds and crystallizes in the developing child between the ages of three and five. During this period, or Oedipal phase, the child craves extraordinary closeness with the same-sex parent and seeks to eliminate the opposite-sex parent as a rival. This triangular development is resolved through renunciation of these wishes and their repression by identifying with the same-sex parent in the formation of conscience and the superego. When unresolved, the competitiveness or rivalry with the same-sex parent, and especially with subsequent derivative transference figures (or the obvious anxious avoidance of competitiveness) sustains the oedipal or competitive character structure, theoretically fueled by castration anxiety in its derivative sense as the threat of punishment. The corresponding development in girls is identified as the Electra complex.

OEDIPUS COMPLEX, NEGATIVE These are instances where the child will admire the same-sex parent and feel an aversion to the opposite-sex parent. Grandiosity or surety is promoted in the identification with the same-sex parent. Such grandiosity acts as the person's characterological engine, as a way of establishing and maintaining the negative oedipal arrangement. It is thought that in this way the attitudes of the opposite-sex parent are held in check, presumably because of the sense that this opposite-sex parent tyrannically insists on controlling the individual and all circumstances. Thus such tyrannical control needs to be nullified for psychosexual development to proceed normally. Negative oedipal feelings are usually seen in highly intelligent children as the way these children manage to safeguard their psychosexual development.

OFF TARGET WORK In psychoanalytic treatment, this refers to the patient's references to people other than the therapist, and to the therapist's interpretations based upon such off target references. See On target work.

OLFACTORY REFERENCE SYNDROME A hallucinatory experience of foul or strange odor.

OMNIPOTENCE Equivalent to megalomania and the sense of omniscience. The person considers the inner signal far more important than external reality signals and thus fortifies self-esteem through the belief in self-importance and self-correctness in all judgments. In extreme form it can be delusional, as in the belief that internal wishes in the form of thoughts can influence the real world. This sort of thinking is a denial, even a renunciation of the reality principle that would necessarily force the subject to realistically confront everyday frustrations and failures. Characterologically, omnipotence is seen in narcissistic disorders and is referred to as the early infantile oceanic feeling. Such individuals seek to erase tension-producing stimuli because these cause doubt, and the omnipotence requires the avoidance and finally the erasure of any doubt. Thus everything needs to be ego-syntonic and not ego-alien, and hence omnipotence is also the fuel for magical thinking. This essentially means that anything that is new and not harmonious with the needs of such an individual, will be rejected. Because such individuals believe that one's wishes should automatically be gratified, poor judgment obtains, leading to a variety of failures and disappointments—results that were precisely and originally avoided. Seen also in narcissistic personalities. See Winnicott, D. W.

ONANISM Refers either to masturbation or to the interruption of sexual intercourse.

ONOMATOPOESIS Equivalent to neologistic word rhymes. Seen in schizophrenic patients who rhyme on the basis of sound associations or associate to a sound and then rhyme in an inexact manner, but in a way that is close to the sound.

ON TARGET WORK In psychoanalysis, on target work refers to the transference interpretations made by the therapist to the patient regarding the patient's feelings about the therapist. Off target work refers to transference interpretations made that do not directly refer to patient in relation to therapist.

ONTOGENY Meaning either biological development during the life span or psychic development, as, for example, either in the Freudian model of oral, anal, phallic, and oedipal development or with respect to any other paradigm of psychological development such as Erikson's psychosocial stages.

ONTOLOGICAL ANXIETY An existential observation regarding one's tension about "being." Further developed by Rollo May.

OPERANT CONDITIONING Process of learning or changing behavior that occurs as a function of the consequences of the behavior (e.g., rewarding behavior change in a child). Idea developed by B. F. Skinner. See Reinforcement; Shaping.

OPERANT CONDITIONING THERAPY Approach, developed by the psychologist B. F. Skinner, in which rewards are utilized to reinforce new behavior. See Reinforcement; Skinner, B. F.

OPPOSITE, REVERSAL INTO THE Defending against libidinous instinct generates a reflexive effect of turning the aim of the instinct into its opposite. This nullifies any prospect of the original instinct fulfilling its aim. It is the change in an impulse, for example, in active to passive, even though the aim of the impulse remains the same.

OPPOSITIONAL DISORDER A condition seen in children who protest, have temper tantrums, insist on getting what they want when they want it (difficulty in delaying gratification), are argumentative, and constantly test boundaries and limits. May be demonstrated on the Rorschach Test by responses that include reversals of figure and ground, in the use of spaces on the blots as foreground perceptions. Similar to conduct disorder.

OPTIMAL DISTANCE A concept utilized in the relational psychotherapies and self psychology. It is a tuning into the patient's comfort zone, or optimal space, and therefore implies accurate empathy on the part of the therapist. Essentially, it refers to an adaptive optimal distance during any developmental stage such as, for example, the proper distance between subject and object in the oedipal phase of development. Optimal distance also implies the idea of optimal responsiveness, as exposited by Howard Bacal.

ORAL-AGGRESSIVE OR ORAL-SADISTIC In psychoanalytic understanding, an early stage of development referring to an oral biting phase that is then displaced or sublimated into envy and exploitative behavior as chief characteristics of the personality.

ORAL CHARACTER A personality disposition of one who is fixated at the oral stage and displays characteristics of excessive optimism and pessimism, moodiness and elation, generosity and greed, demandingness, dependency, and impatience.

ORAL EROTIC Pleasure associated with the mouth.

ORALITY Refers to derivatives of the oral or first phase of psychosexual development. Traits of orality include generosity and receptivity to others and presumably imply that the person is wishful of being replied to in kind. The qualities of orality may also encompass greedy, demanding, incorporative and dependent traits. Orality is postulated as one basis for the appearance of manic-depressive pathology.

ORAL STAGE The first stage of psychosexual development, from birth to two years, in which the mouth is the chief source of attachment and libidinal, instinctual, or individual gratification for the child. As such it is within the closeness embodied in this stage that the child establishes a symbiotic relationship with its caretaker, which, if reliably fulfilling, leads later to the successful emergence of individuation.

ORBITAL PREFRONTAL FUNCTION OF THE BRAIN See Personality / character disorder.

ORGANIC ANXIETY SYNDROME Anxiety attacks and / or panic attacks that are organically based.

ORGANIC BRAIN SYNDROME Disturbance in thinking and behavior based upon physical brain trauma. Disturbances of concentration, cognitive abilities, abstract thinking are examples of impairment of such mental functioning. Behaviorally, poor frustration tolerance and subsequent sudden impulsive behavior is also seen.

ORGANIC MENTAL DISORDERS In the psychiatric nomenclature, such disorders and symptoms include senile dementia, delirium, delusional disorders, hallucinations.

ORGASM A sexual excitation that reaches a crescendo or climax, usually as a result of sexual stimulation. The physical satisfactory completion of sexual intercourse.

ORIENTATION The status of an individual's knowledge and awareness of his or her person, location, and temporal experience. It is tapped in the psychiatric clinical examination that assesses the subject's sense of person, place, and time. Such a person can accurately identify others, can locate the self, and can name the day, week, year, and location at which the examination is taking place or where the person is residing.

ORIENTATION, DOUBLE Referring to a person who can function normally in a variety of ways, yet still maintain a pathological delusion, as, for example, of some sort of grandiose sense of self. Also referred to as an encapsulated delusion or a dysmorphophobia.

ORIGINAL RESPONSE See Rorschach Test.

ORTHOPSYCHIATRY Concerned with the conventional parameters of mental health as well as with the deviations from such parameters.

ORTHRIOGENESIS The recapitulation of the ego's full development each time upon waking. Essentially a return or restoration of the person's entire cathected repertoire, which is generally reputed to be lost during sleep. Attributed to Federn.

OSSIFICATION, CHARACTEROLOGICAL Rigidity of behavioral patterns that are clinically considered to be character traits.

OUTPATIENT Those individuals who are no longer hospitalized but make repeated visits to the hospital clinic for treatment continuity and therapeutic services.

OVERCOMPENSATION A popular term, which, as a clinical definition, is actually a redundancy. Generally, compensatory behavior is the defense of choice of those individuals who are either depressed and defending against depression or who experience the self as grossly inadequate or inferior. Such individuals utilize compensatory fantasy and behaviors to suppress negative self-evaluation in favor of more agreeable notions and evidence of self-worth. When used to counteract depression, the compensation becomes a defense that services a pattern of characterological responses called character trait patterns. When utilized as a defense against feelings of inferiority, compensation may be considered an emotion defense against event-related despairing feelings. The term *compensation* also corresponds to the language of Adlerian psychotherapy concerning a person's striving for ego elevation.

OVERDETERMINATION A concept popularized in working with dreams within a psychoanalytic framework. The idea is that the manifest dream (the dream remembered, or referred to as "the dream from above") is a function of several factors and contains a multilayered motive formation that, when unraveled, will reveal the multifaceted, multilayered, or overdetermined nature of the dream. Thus there is more than a single interpretation that can be applied to various aspects of the dream, based upon psychosexual level or even upon intrapsychic considerations of id / superego conflict. The idea of overdetermination also applies to other products of the psyche such as symptoms. See Dream theory, Freudian.

OVERINCLUSIVENESS In schizophrenic thinking, associative disturbances can include the combination of layers of meaning into one concept so that meanings become simultaneously overabstract (lose specificity) and also overly concrete (each element of the thought being quite specific, but not necessarily directly related to other elements).

P

PAIN, ECSTATIC Essentially reflective of a masochistic position in which a person will tend to sacrifice for others or spend inordinate energy on self-projects and, in addition, is willing to suffer unpleasant conditions in the extreme—all in the service of whatever the project. In such cases the person frequently martyrs the self and experiences what is known as "no good deed will go unpunished." Originally called a hunger for excitement, the ecstatic pain phenomenon is really part of the obsessive-compulsive syndrome, with a strong masochistic element. The masochistic element is ostensibly derived from a need to expiate guilt because of a hypothesized store of repressed anger toward a historical figure—parent or parent surrogate. This presumed repressed anger toward such a figure, as well as its subsequent guilt, is usually a chronic condition beginning in childhood and then acted out throughout life. It becomes the birth of masochism, housed within obsessive-compulsive parameters, based upon the person's expiation need. See Masochism; Obsessive-compulsive.

PAIN DISORDER Excessive pain in a specific body locations attributed to stress or a particular psychological problem. See Psychogenic pain disorder; Somatoform disorders.

PAIN MANAGEMENT Use of behavior conditioning techniques to better manage pain.

PAIRING GROUP See Assumption group.

PALEOLOGIC THINKING Equivalent to paralogical or syncretistic thinking, essentially meaning correlational thinking in which the person links two events, which may occur serially or simultaneously, that are then interpreted as cause and effect. The thinking is said to be concrete and, in extreme form, to reflect psychotic thinking. Therefore, paleologic thinking ushers in the high probability of the presence of delusional feelings. Associated with this cluster of meanings (paleologic, paralogical, and syncretistic thinking) is parataxic distortion (introduced by Sullivan), essentially referring to distortions of the transference.

PAN-ANXIETY A cardinal feature in former psychiatric nosology, the main characteristic of the diagnosis being that the person functions with anxiety in virtually all facets of life. The diagnosis is in the psychotic category, in which the person is quite ambulatory but permeated with tension. Hence the diagnosis of pseudoneurotic schizophrenia, with the person appearing neurotically radiated with anxiety, while beneath lies the psychotic disorganization.

PANIC, PREPSYCHOTIC A precursor to the full flowering of a schizophrenic diagnosis, in which the person degrades the self to the point of self-humiliation. Still, in this stage of the process leading up to the schizophrenic diagnosis the person temporarily retains reasonable cognitive functioning.

PANIC DISORDER In panic, the person is overwhelmed, and the experience of the panic (along with its feelings of terror and dread) can lead to a sense of depersonalization. Clinically, those individuals with panic frequently describe themselves as "going crazy." In the anxiety disorder, the person experiences a particularly distressing amount of tension but can still cope. Unlike the anxiety disorder, the panic disorder entirely disables the person. Panic disorders generally are Axis I *DSM*–classified as variations of anxiety disorders.

PANKSEPP, JAAK (1943–). Estonian-born American physiological psychologist. Pioneer of the field of neuropsychoanalysis. Interested in the investigation of the mind (the cognitive brain) and behavior so as to more profoundly understand the nature of emotion. Panksepp identified primary emotional phenotypes, the assumption being that understanding the emotional neural level will shed light on human emotional disorders. Studied the neurobiological nature of emotional processes as these relate to psychotherapeutic practice. In his work on the anatomy of emotions, Panksepp has suggested that basic emotions are organized via long-axoned, sensory-motor command systems that interconnect higher and lower functions of the brain. He identified a foraging-expectancy circuitry, a rage circuitry, a fear circuitry, and a panic circuitry. See Dopaminergic "seeking" system.

PARADOX, NEUROTIC In psychoanalytic theory, the paradox is understood as neurotic behavior that persists, even though such neurotic behavior undermines the person's relationships and distorts other aspects of life. This paradox is resolved, however, through Freud's notion that in the psyche no wish will be denied. In this way, the neurosis persists because within the neurosis lies the facet of the personality that generates psychological symptoms. Thus, according to Freud, we love our symptoms because they are our wishes fully realized—albeit perversely or neurotically; that is, through a symptom that serves as a symbol of the wish. Hence the paradox regarding the persistence of even a painful neurosis is solved, because the love of our neurosis contains psychically, albeit symbolically, gratified wishes in the form of the symptom. See Symptom.

PARADOXICAL INTENTION (PI) A paradigmatic technique that fosters greater anxiety in phobic individuals as a way to ultimately and presumably undermine the phobic response. Related to the counterphobic concept. Essentially the subject is challenged to do what is feared.

PARADOXICAL TECHNIQUES See Paradoxical therapy.

PARADOXICAL THERAPY The patient is encouraged to do exactly what the symptom addresses and what the treatment is designed to eliminate. It is also known as strategic therapy. It goes along with the pathology rather than contradicting it, then applying strategic intervention to adjust the patient's interpretation of the problem. Introduced by Jay Haley and Richard Rabkin and utilized in family therapy.

PARALOGIA Logic that becomes contaminated by the constant displacement of synonyms and is then evidenced as poor reasoning during verbal interaction with others.

PARALOGICAL THINKING See Syncretistic thinking.

PARALYSIS, HYSTERICAL Equivalent to conversion hysteria in which a limb can become functionally paralyzed with no apparent physical or organic cause. Initially treated by Charcot and Freud in the late nineteenth century. See Hysteria.

PARAMETER, PSYCHOANALYTIC A reference to the boundary permitted between therapist and patient in order to keep the transference possibilities with respect to interpretation objective and uncontaminated. Also refers to the particular therapeutic arrangement regarding the nature of treatment as it is modified from classical form.

PARANOIA Referring essentially to delusion-prone mental functioning. Freud related paranoia to a defense against homosexual urges—to wit: "I love him" becomes "I hate him," which in turn becomes "He hates me."

PARANOIA, INVOLUTIONAL The paranoid aspect of involutional melancholia. See Involutional psychosis.

PARANOID ANXIETY Concern with a possible attack by projected objects seen as bad.

PARANOID DISORDER A delusional disorder. Personality vicissitudes include the use of defined projection mechanisms, heightened critical scrutiny to protect the self from anything that differs from existing internal psychic organization, a corresponding suspiciousness, and a highly sensitized vigilance to the immediate environment. Delusions are either grandiose or persecutory. Variations include

shared paranoid system—between parent and child, called a folie à deux;

encapsulated paranoia condition—in which general functioning is normal except for that one defined arena contaminated by delusion. Classic Freudian etiology speculates that the genesis of the paranoid condition is underpinned by a homosexual orientation.

PARANOID DISORDER, SHARED See Shared paranoid disorder.

PARANOID PERSONALITY Traits such as stubbornness, jealousy, criticality, and envy characterize such a person. Considered to be a character disorder that diagnostically resides within *DSM* nomenclature as a personality disorder category and considered nonpsychotic.

PARANOID-SCHIZOID POSITION See Klein, Melanie.

PARANOID SCHIZOPHRENIA A psychotic condition and best known of the schizophrenias. In all forms of schizophrenia, a thinking disorder characterizes the diagnosis. In the paranoid form, delusions of persecution or grandiosity are characteristic. Historically, the basic schizophrenias were termed as follows.

Simple—a cardinal characteristic is flat affect.
Hebephrenic—silliness, grimacing, and inappropriate laughing.
Catatonic—waxy flexibility and excitement is seen.
Paranoid—persecutory or grandiose delusions and hallucinations.

Other paranoid diagnoses have included:

Acute—sudden onset with a decent prognosis.
Ambulatory—encapsulated, so that the person can function.
Episodic—event-related disturbance.
Pseudoneurotic—person radiated with anxiety (pan-anxiety), showing neuroticlike behavior above and schizophrenic / paranoid elements, below.

Historically, the presence of all Bleuhler's four As satisfied the criteria for the diagnosis of a thinking disorder. These are

Associative disturbance—language and communication contamination.
Ambivalence—inability to be decisive.
Affect—flat or otherwise disturbed.
Autism—meaning highly idiosyncratic and unrealistic thinking.

Contemporary criteria for the diagnosis of schizophrenia also include an assessment of the patient's orientation to time, place, and person as well as a fuller content analysis of the clinical picture. See Orientation.

PARANOID STATE Bizarre associations absent. Delusions present, but are not systematized as they would be in schizophrenia. Hallucinations absent.

PARANOSIC GAIN See Gain, primary.

PARAPATHIC PROVISO A form of syncretistic or correlational thinking in which the person will assume an obsessional ruminating position, as, for example, that remaining ill will assure the health of a loved one. Also referred to as neurotic proviso and made popular by Stekel as well as Adler.

PARAPHILIA A characterization utilized in the psychiatric nomenclature to reflect sexual deviation including exhibitionism, fetishism, pedophilia, and transvesticism.

PARAPRAXIS A Freudian concept devoted to the understanding of unconscious acts such as forgetfulness or slips of the tongue.

PARAPSYCHOLOGY The ostensible possessing or research of presumed extrasensory ability such as telepathy and clairvoyance.

PARASEXUALITY Early development of an interest in all things sexually perverse.

PARASOMNIA Reference to disturbed sleep. The major parasomnias include

Nightmare—dream content that awakens the dreamer. See Nightmare.

REM disturbed sleep—disturbed dream sleep.

Sleepwalking—walking during sleep with no awareness of the event.

Sleep paralysis—inability to move either when entering or exiting sleep.

Sleep terror—awakening in terror during non-REM (NREM) sleep, that is, nondream sleep.

See See Narcolepsy; Sleep disorders.

PARATAXIC See Distortion, parataxic.

PARRICIDE Murder of the father. Usually interpreted in relation to the Oedipus complex.

PARTIAL ADJUSTMENTS A subtle observation by Sullivan that focuses on the period immediately preceding an acute traumatic event (prepsychotic), where the subject begins to utilize a host of defenses to ward off anxiety. These defensive maneuvers include evasions, rationalizations, and a variety of compensatory strategies.

PARTIAL HOSPITALIZATION Usually refers to day-hospital visits or weekend visits to the outpatient treatment center of the hospital.

PART OBJECT RELATIONS Frequently referred to in a sexual context in which the person seeks sexual gratification from a focus on only specific parts of the body and not on the whole person. Also referred to as "partialism" and, in obsessional form, considered to be a perversion. With respect to relationships, rather than leading to an object constancy, such a part object focus solely concerns the subject's own need for gratification. Seen as a defense against development of any primary or permanent relationship.

PASSIVE-AGGRESSIVE PERSONALITY In the general mental health nomenclature, considered to be in the category of a character or personality disorder. The passive-aggressive person engages in behavior designed to invoke anger or rage in the object (the other person). Historically, the passive-aggressive personality was seen to be composed of three types:

Passive type—in which behaviors of delay frustrate the other, thus achieving the passive-aggressive goal.

Aggressive type—in which arrogance or overentitled insistence by the subject also achieves the goal of invoking anger in the other.

Dependent type—in which the subject becomes exceedingly reliant on another and in this way again invokes anger in the other because of the inherent burden implicit in such dependence.

In all cases of personality or character disorders, the particular behavioral pattern is not interfered with or modified by anxiety, because the purpose of such characterological organization (in this case, passive-aggressive), is to bind anxiety rather than to feel it. Victory over or defense against the object is always the passive-aggressive aim. This is accomplished by frustrating/and or burdening the object. The basic underlying motive or force of such a person is generated by ambivalence and negativism toward the object. Features of the subject's personality include procrastination, stubbornness, and even forgetfulness. Also referred to as negative personality disorder.

PASSIVITY Classic behind the line activity and equivalent to withdrawal from engaging in initiating behaviors. Front of the line is a doing place. Behind the line is a place of passivity and rumination—a not-doing place. See Line, The.

PASTORAL COUNSELING Especially useful for people of faith. Pastoral counselors offer guidance and provide a venue for people seeking help for any number of life's challenges. Pastoral counselors are usually trained in psychotherapeutic methods.

PATERNALISM In a clinical sense, refers to control of another in the guise of expressing interest and care.

PATHO Essentially meaning disease, dis-ease, or suffering.

PATHOCURE The inhibition of any neurosis in the face of a severe biologically based disease. It is the opposite of pathoneurosis, which is the promotion of neurosis based on the onset of a biological disease.

PATHOGNOMONIC The salient or symptom-identifying characteristic of a specific diagnosis. The major variable that characterizes the diagnosis.

PATHOGRAPHY OR PATHOBIOGRAPHY Using biographical data to augment understanding of the subject—in particular, with reference to psychopathology.

PATHOLOGY Referring to the nature of disease.

PATHONEUROSIS See Pathocure.

PATTERN, SPECIFIC DYNAMIC Related to the key psychodynamic of a psychosomatic disorder. Coined by Franz Alexander.

PAVLOV, IVAN (1849–1936). Russian physiologist and physician who studied experimental neuroses in animals. Considered the father of classical conditioning, his work later inspired the originators of behavior therapy.

PEDERASTY Anal intercourse between and a man and a boy.

PEDOPHILIA Refers to the sexual attraction to young boys or girls.

PEEPING TOM Refers to voyeurism.

PENIS ENVY In psychoanalysis, refers to girls having regret about not having, and rather wanting, a penis. In heterosexual men, can also be seen in symbolic form in the obsession with the female breast—that is, the large breast—insofar as the large breast represents the large penis so that in men such possessive interest generates feelings of adequacy.

PENIS PRIDE Melanie Klein's phrase for the boy's compensatory sense of ascendancy or superiority.

PERCEPTANALYSIS Zygmunt Piotrowski's system of Rorschach analysis.

PERLS, FRITZ (1893–1970). Friedrich Salomon Perls. German-born American psychiatrist who was the most influential practitioner and theoretician of Gestalt therapy. See Gestalt therapy.

PERPLEXITY, VAGUE Seen in patients with organic brain disorder. Patient will be mentally confused, and cognitive faculties will be affected. Drowsiness is also seen frequently.

PERSEVERATION Behavior or verbal output that is persistent—as in the continuous repetition of a phrase or an act. Seen in patients with organic brain syndrome and in schizophrenic thinking as related to disturbance of association.

PERSONA That part of the person's attitude and emotional posture that either faithfully reflects the person's authenticity or that promotes artifice. Mask. Used by Jung.

PERSONALITY Sustained patterns of behavior, attitudes, cognitive organization, and emotional tone that characterizes an individual's style, thereby giving that person a distinctive and recognizable configuration. In clinical usage, personality is roughly equivalent to character—in terms of character structure—so that personality disorder as a diagnostic category is the same as that of character disorder.

PERSONALITY, AS IF See As if personality.

PERSONALITY / CHARACTER DISORDER Axis II diagnoses of the *DSM* nomenclature are the character or personality disorders. These are patterns of personality referred to as characterological states that form a syndrome in which a consistent set of behaviors are reflexively expressed, not guided by tensions or considerations as to whether such behaviors could be self-defeating. Therefore, in this personality disorder category, anxiety is presumed to be bound. Correspondingly, in the absence of experienced anxiety, the subject is not sufficiently assisted by an internal warning signal to support better judgment with respect to behavior. In this sense, shifting to a more mature stance requires the attempt in psychotherapy to, so to speak, loosen the anxiety so that it may be experienced, thereby bringing into existence such an internal warning signal. In the domain of neuropsychoanalysis, and according to Schore, all characterological psychopathology implicates an altered orbital prefrontal function of the brain. The complement of these Axis II disorders and their salient characteristics include the following types:

Antisocial—poor sense of boundaries, delinquency.
Avoidant—sensitivity to criticism, social inhibition.
Borderline—relationship instability, thin stimulus-barrier.
Compulsive—focus on perfection and orderliness.
Dependent—separation fear, submissive and clinging behavior.
Histrionic—excessive emotionality, attention seeking.
Narcissistic—grandiosity, need for adoration, lacking empathy.
Paranoid—distrust, suspicion, and a critical attitude.
Passive-aggressive—motive is to satisfy anger by frustrating the object.
Schizoid—detachment, restriction of emotion.
Schizotypal—discomfort with relationships, odd behavior.

In addition, other such personality disorders include:

Cyclothymic—cycles of hypomania and depression.
Masochistic—inviting punishment, and/or pain.
Posttraumatic—reliving of previous trauma—either picturing it and/or feeling it.

Sadistic—seeking to inflict pain.

Transient situational—symptoms occur to difficult situations.

Among the many contributors to the understanding of character or personality disorders are included Blatt, Burry, Corsini, Josephs, Reich, and Shapiro.

PERSONALITY TYPE A phrase associated with the designation of typologies. Jung's extraversion and introversion or Sheldon's body / psyche types are examples.

PESONIFICATION Attributing to another various values and emotions, as in the objectification in which the object is infused with particular attributes.

PERVASIVE DEVELOPMENTAL DISORDERS In the DSM nosology, these disorders, as well as sample symptoms, include

Autistic disorder—characterized by social fragmentation, idiosyncratic behavior, and withdrawal, along with a host of developmental arrests. See Autism.

Asperger's disorder—compromised emotional reciprocity in high-level autism. Ability to function at a high level of abstraction is seen. See Asperger's syndrome.

Attention-deficit / hyperactivity disorder—a disorder of concentration and reduced attention span that includes impulsivity and hyperactivity. See Attention-deficit/ hyperactivity disorder.

Childhood disintegrative disorder—loss of most socialized capacity before the age of ten. See Childhood disintegrative disorder.

Rett's disorder—loss of previously developed motor and language development along with stereotyped movements between ages five months to thirty months. See Rett's disorder.

PERVERSION Abnormality from the norm. Clinically, usually means sexual atypicality or that which is considered sexually impermissible and therefore to be hidden.

PHALLIC A psychological reference to the penis. In psychoanalysis, referring to the psychosexual stage preceding the oedipal period, following the anal period.

PHALLIC CHARACTER A person who is interested in the compensatory display of power and seeks admiration or appreciation of qualities thought to be special. Essentially refers to pride in the penis and, in a derivative sense, the desire to be exhibitionistic and assertive, as well as expressing an inclination for striving.

PHANTOM LIMB After the loss of a limb, the person's experiencing the sensation of its presence, its existence. The phantom limb sensation is most likely to occur when a limb is lost suddenly, through accident or surgical amputation, and is unlikely when the loss occurs gradually, as in leprosy. These factors affecting the phantom limb sensation are thought to reflect the brain's propensity to adapt gradually to body changes and its inability to assimilate abrupt change all at once.

PHANTOM LOVER Usually seen in women. The fantasy is of being loved by an idealized figure (usually a man). Psychologically, this syndrome is compensatory in nature, frequently to a sense of narcissistic injury, which is presumably derived from a history of affectional deprivation.

PHASE SHIFT Referring to the sleep disorder in which the day and night seem to be reversed so that sleepiness occurs when wakefulness would be expected. See Sleep disorders.

PHENOMENOLOGICAL REALITY See Morita therapy.

PHENOMENOLOGY A focus on experience, and equivalent to existential psychology. See May, Rollo.

PHENOTYPE Developmental changes the individual undergoes as a result of external environmental factors. Contrasts with genotype—changes occurring despite environmental experience.

PHENYLKETONURIA An inherited disorder that can affect intelligence quotient, but can be detected early on by a simple urine test and cured through diet.

PHEROMONE One's odor affecting the response of another same-species organism.

PHILOBAT In Balint's system refers to a person who is a thrill seeker but is never really attached to others. See Balint, Michael.

PHLEGMATIC TYPE Galen's term for an apathetic type.

PHOBIA An irrational and intense fear of a particular object or situation, usually leading to significant restriction of everyday functioning. Considered to be an Axis I *DSM* disorder along the spectrum of anxiety disorders. A sample of phobia categories include:

Agoraphobia—can be life threatening, as in the end result of the fear of open spaces that leads to the extreme fear of even leaving the bed. See Agoraphobia.
Claustrophobia—fear of being closed in. See Claustrophobia.
Polyphobia—ubiquitous fears.
School phobia—a frequent phobia seen in children or adolescents. Usually associated with separation anxiety from a primary caregiver. It is thought that the extreme anxiety covers anger toward this same object.
Simple phobia—fear of any specific object (e.g., snake or injections).
Social phobia—intense apprehension of social situations, considered to be a function of early parental disregard.

Phobias can include death fears, hypochondriacal fears, and any number of other specific loci of fear. According to Freudian precepts, such a symptom would imply that behind the fear is the wish, so that the phobic symptom is some perverse or neurotic disguise for the wish. Thus, it is debatable whether the emotion of fear is the actual unconscious basis of any phobia. According to Kellerman, as it is in any symptom, repressed anger toward a specific person is the real basis of any symptom, so that repressed anger may be the true underlying emotion culprit in all phobias. In cognitive behavior therapy, commonly treated by relaxation training and anti-awfulizing about the feared situation, followed by repeated exposure to the feared stimulus using the various coping skills learned in treatment. See Anger; Symptom.

PHONOLOGY The sound morphology of language.

PHRENOLOGY Discredited nineteenth-century study of personality and mental function on the basis of the configuration of the skull.

PIAGET, JEAN (1896–1980). Swiss psychologist specializing in the study of the cognitive structure in children. Influential in the field of developmental psychology. Studied the evolution of human intelligence and proposed a system of stages of cognitive development:

The sensorimotor stage—birth to two years. Children experience the world through movement and senses.
The preoperational stage—two to seven years. Acquisition of motor skills.
The concrete operational stage—seven to eleven years. Logical thinking appears.
The formal operational stage—after age eleven. Crystallization of abstract reasoning.

PIGEM'S QUOTIENT An aspect of the mental examination that aims, through projective questions, to elicit from the patient responses that reveal what the patient would do to change the status quo.

PIOTROWSKI, ZYGMUNT A. (1904–1985). European-born American psychologist best known for his Rorschach interpretive system called Perceptanalysis.

PLACEBO Subtle influence on an individual that occurs because the person has a conscious expectation that either a procedure or medication will result in a cure. In this sense, the element of suggestion is strongly implicated in the entire process. In addition, the use of a placebo invites the subject's cooperation so that, even among people diagnosed with an obsessive disorder, the placebo's inherent suggestibility factor and the subject's positive anticipation increases effectiveness.

PLAY THERAPY A technique of understanding the child's communication through its play with any number of objects. This enables the therapist to relate to the child in the absence of requiring sophisticated verbal communication.

PLEASURE-PAIN PRINCIPLE In psychoanalytic thinking, the pleasure-pain principle explains the individual's desire to reduce painful stimuli and therefore attain pleasure. The discharge of drives also affords pleasure. The main derivative expression of the pleasure principle is in instinctual release and finally in the appearance of wishes.

PLUTCHIK, ROBERT (1928–2006). American psychologist. Chiefly known for his classic influential text on the psychoevolutionary theory of emotion. Promoted use of the circumplex grid to illustrate relationships between primary emotions and a variety of other clinical phenomena. His coedited five-volume work on emotion comprised the first repository source for the scientific and clinical organization of emotion theory. Authored texts on emotion in relation to biological foundations, psychotherapy, ego defenses, and personality. His scientific volume on the *Foundations of Experimental Research* became one of the standard resources for understanding methodology in the approach to psychological laboratory work that is also applicable to clinical studies.

POLARITY Referring to opposites. In Freudian terms, three polarities account for the underpinning of the psyche.

Active-passive—a concept of the calibration of the psyche's confrontation with the demands of reality, with "active" corresponding to masculinity and "passive" corresponding to femininity. Contamination or psychosexual difficulties occur presumably when the correlation of such correspondences significantly decrease.

Pleasure-pain—focus on either release or blockage of instinctual pressures or tension, with the release correlating to increase of pleasure and decrease of pain, and blockage correlating to increase of pain and decrease of pleasure.

Subject-object—essentially an epigenetic conception that considers the subject's operation and management of instinctual tension within the subject-object context.

POLLYANNA Equivalent to consistent optimism. The defense of denial accompanies this proclivity.

POLYANDRY Opposite of polygamy, that is, one woman possessing several men.

POLYMORPHOUS PERVERSE Indulging in sexual behavior with respect to including a wide variety of sexual partners that obey no usual expectations, such as same-sex partners, infantile fantasy sex, or any number of other sexual variations.

POLYPHAGIA Equivalent to bulimia; also means gluttony.

POLYSOMNOGRAM (PSM) The sleep profile of results of a battery of sleep tests while the subject is asleep. Used in sleep laboratories in the study of various sleep disorders. Includes results of the electroencephalogram.

PONTINE REGIONS According to Panksepp, in the domain of neuropsychoanalysis, the drives are a series of basic emotions anchored in these regions. Such emotions include anger, caring, fear, seeking play, and sadness.

POPULAR RESPONSE Those percept responses on the Rorschach that are frequently produced (seen).

PORNOGRAPHY Prurient sexual interest.

POSITION/TRANCE DISORDER Historically considered a dissociative disorder in which the subject feels possessed and is therefore absorbed with the internal signal at the expense of a decent measure of reality testing. The dissociated state is seen in the subject's altered consciousness.

POSITIVE PSYCHOLOGY See Seligman, Martin.

POSITIVE REINFORCEMENT See Reinforcement.

POSTAMBIVALENT STAGE The stage at which a person can develop a relationship and is considered with respect to the readiness for object love.

POSTGRADUATE CENTER FOR MENTAL HEALTH See Wolberg, Lewis R.

POSTHYPNOTIC SUGGESTION During hypnosis, a suggestion is made that is to be acted upon posthypnosis.

POSTPARTUM PSYCHOSIS Usually seen in women immediately after giving birth and frequently associated with postpartum depression.

POSTSCHIZOPHRENIC DEPRESSION May follow an acute schizophrenic process and considered restitutive, especially when the depression predated the schizophrenic process and was disguised by it.

POSTTRAUMATIC STRESS DISORDER Future emotional effect of a catastrophic or highly stressful event. Responses consist of intrusive thoughts, recurrent nightmares, startle reaction, anxiety attacks, and cognitive difficulties such as impaired concentration and attention span. An Axis I example of an anxiety disorder in *DSM* nosology.

POTENCY Referring to the ability to perform adequately. Clinically, refers to a man's ability to perform in sexual contact.

PPO Preferred Provider Organization. A health care delivery system.

PRECOCITY Exceptional ability in a child, occurring earlier than what would be conventionally expected.

PRECOGNITION Equivalent to ostensible or so-called extrasensory perception in that there is an assumed ability to foretell the thinking of others or to predict future events.

PRECONSCIOUS Part of Freud's topographical theory of the conscious, preconscious, and unconscious. In the preconscious, memories can relatively easily be brought into consciousness. See Freud, Sigmund.

PREDISPOSITION Clinically, meaning a greater readiness to express or display certain traits based upon genetic givens.

PREGENITAL Referring to the psychosexual phase preceding mature development.

PREMATURE EJACULATION Referring to the male's preemptive ejaculation or excited seminal emission. Can cause the partner to feel rejected, perhaps angry, or even abandoned. Other than any biological etiology, this difficulty can be attributed to a quasi-conscious tension (apprehension) with a more psychologically significant suppressed underlying anger, coalescing in a general difficulty with commitment in relationships. Also thought theoretically to reflect either an overcompliance with gratifying the partner, thus the loss of control in a preemptory moment, or, alternatively, a passive-aggressive act denying pleasure on a transference level to the partner as, hypothetically, a mother figure.

PREMENSTRUAL TENSION STATE Also known as PMS and referring to a woman's sense of her impending period, which can cause her anxiety, discomfort, frustration, and general dis-ease. This tension syndrome dissipates with the arrival of the period.

PREMORBID The general personality immediately preceding the onset of pathology. The pathological morbidity becomes the altered personality.

PREOEDIPAL Referring to the psychosexual stages of oral, anal, and phallic that precede the oedipal stage. See Freud, Sigmund.

PREPSYCHOTIC Referring to the personality preceding a psychotic process.

PREPSYCHOTIC PERSONALITY An individual's nonpsychotic personality (the type of the character structure) before psychosis appears.

PREPUBERTAL Referring to the period preceding puberty.

PREREFLECTIVE UNCONSCIOUS From an intersubjective understanding, this refers to the invariant organizing stimuli outside a person's awareness that can influence the person's experience. See Intersubjectivity theory; Stolorow, Robert.

PRESENILE Referring to the stage preceding senility.

PRESSURE OF IDEAS Also referred to as thought pressure. Seen in schizophrenic patients who feel vulnerable to the ideas of others and then ascribe the thoughts that enter their minds to the influence of these others. Understood as a projective identification characteristic mostly of paranoid schizophrenic patients, but also seen in other schizophrenic diagnoses. Attributed possibly to the person's "thin-stimulus barrier" and obsessive rigidity of the ego.

PRIAPIC DRIVE Phallic assertive intention.

PRIAPISM A variation of erectile dysfunction in which the erect penis continues to remain erect. Rather than a function of sexual excitation, it is more a biologically painful dysfunction.

PRIDE SYSTEM Horney's concept of the person's extreme estimate of the self, from idealizing the self to assessing the negative self.

PRIMACY ZONE See Zone, erogenous.

PRIMAL SCENE During childhood, for the first time, observing the sexual act of parents. In classical psychoanalytic thinking, presumed to be etiologically important in the future organization of the psyche and manifested in any number of psychopathological patterns.

PRIMAL THERAPY A much disputed experiential therapy proposed by Arthur Janov (1924–), an American psychologist. In this approach, patients need to reexperience their original pain in order to achieve favorable therapeutic results. Connecting past events to the present is seen as the attempt to connect meaning to emotion. Three levels of consciousness are accessed in primal therapy and proposed to represent the multidimensional nature of repression. In this sense, repression can be a physical, emotional, or intellectual aspect of consciousness. Janov is best known for his volume *The Primal Scream*.

PRIMAL TRAUMA See Infantile trauma.

PRIMARY MATERNAL PREOCCUPATION A special psychological condition of the mother for several weeks before and after the birth of the baby. The mother withdraws and is preoccupied with the infant. It is a temporary "healthy illness" that presumably heightens the mother's adaptation to the infant's needs.

PRIMARY PROCESS Governed by the pleasure principle, the primary process is primitive cognitive thinking that disregards time and space and contains, on an emotional level, an amorphous bombardment of internal stimuli. It is drive-dominated ideation and can be seen in psychotic speech; as such it demonstrates its lack of concern for logic and reality. Mechanisms of displacement and condensation aggregate images, thoughts, and impulses so that symbolization can be used to interchange meanings. Since the pleasure principle applies to primary process thinking, hallucination is a possible manifestation. The main derivatives of the pleasure principle are wishes and desires that prevail within the deepest infrastructural motivation of the psyche. Primary process as a classic psychoanalytic concept is the material of the latent content of dreams, which translates into the manifest dream through the mechanisms of symbolization, displacement, condensation, and secondary elaboration (the interstitial or connective mechanisms that organize elements of the story line). In contrast, the secondary process is governed by thought and logic and develops later in the maturational process. In the domain of neuropsychoanalysis, primary process is associated with right brain unconscious affective processes. See Dream theory, Freudian; Frontal executive control of mesocortical and mesolimbic "seeking" systems; Right brain emotional processes.

PRIMITIVE MENTAL STATES Mostly referring to schizophrenic thinking. Contributors to this literature include Arieti and Giovacchini.

PRIMITIVIZATION A regression in which hallucination and wish fulfillment replace adequate secondary process and reality testing. Primitivization essentially translates as magical thinking.

PRINCE, MORTON (1854–1929). American psychiatrist best known for his delineation of what has been known as split personality and is now known as dissociative identity disorder. It is a disorder of disassociation. See Dissociative disorders.

PROBLEM, THE HARD See Neuropsychoanalysis.

PRODROMAL Referring to an eventual diagnostic syndrome based upon the presence of precursor symptoms and/or traits.

PROGNOSIS Estimating the possible recovery from an illness. This kind of prediction covers the range of possibility from either good (good chance of recovery) to guarded (poor prognosis).

PROJECTION Attributing qualities that you yourself possess (but are not noticed in the self) to others. These usually consist of negative attributes that are rejected as objectionable. Projection is one among a variety of ego defenses and usually associated with paranoia (especially with respect to delusions of persecution) and also considered an important aspect of the underlying hypothetical dynamic of the paranoid schizophrenic person, who, according to Freud, presumably harbors latent homosexual urges.

PROJECTIVE IDENTIFICATION Seeing qualities of the self in the other that are unconsciously repudiated and then identifying with them. In Klein's view, these disavowed feelings are projected to the analyst, resulting in the patient treating the analyst negatively in order to maintain a measure of control. See Defense mechanisms.

PROJECTIVE PSYCHOLOGY AND DIAGNOSIS During the mid-twentieth century and thereafter, and from a psychodynamic / psychoanalytic vantage point, the Rorschach Test was the premier projective instrument utilized in personality assessment. Some of the luminaries associated with projective psychology included Ainsworth, F. Brown, Exner, B. Klopfer, W. Klopfer, K. Machover, Murray, Ogden, Phillips, Piotrowski, Rorschach, E. Schachtel, D. Shapiro, Sherman, and Smith.

PROJECTIVE TEST BATTERY The conventional projective test battery consists of

Rorschach Test—presentation of ink blots requiring the subject to offer percepts to the blots;
Thematic Apperception Test—presentation of pictures of scenes to which the subject creates a storyline of past, present, and future;
Machover Draw a Person Test—in which the subject is required to draw a person.

Other tests used as material for projective responses include House-Tree-Person, Bender Gestalt, Animal Metaphors, and even some subtests of the Wechsler Intelligence Scales.

PROMISCUITY Indiscriminate and frequent sexual activity.

PROSODY Referring to the variety of elements of speech and vocal expression.

PROTOMASOCHISM The furthest extrapolation of the concept of the death instinct. Related to destruction and sadism and antithetical to the ego.

PRURITUS, PSYCHOGENIC Itching associated with emotional cause and considered to be a psychophysiological reaction.

PSEUDOAGGRESSION Because of a masochistic need to be treated poorly, this person projects a persona of aggression as a way of not seeing the true nature of the masochism. In this sense, the false aggression or pseudoaggression is an acting out insofar as it is an attempt not to know something (the need to be mistreated).

PSEUDOAMNESIA Amnesia that is either feigned or part of a dissociated state.

PSEUDOHALLUCINATION Experiencing a hallucination and understandizing simultaneously that it is not real.

PSEUDOIDENTIFICATION A chameleonlike approach in which the person assumes the attitudes, emotional disposition, and ideas of another in order to avoid conflict.

PSEUDOLOGIA FANTASTICA A symptom of Munchhausen syndrome. Can also be seen in psychopathic individuals who create stories because of a need for continuous external stimulation. It is thought that the person experiences the self as having an impoverished inner life, thereby requiring the creation of such endless external stimulations. Thus it is a fear of silence in the inner life. Also seen in organically damaged individuals. See Munchhausen syndrome.

PSEUDOMANIA Also referred to as shame psychosis and equivalent to an enosiophobia. Here the person is fraught with apprehension about having possibly committed a crime. With some such individuals, even writing something in black and white can be an enormous challenge the person will refuse because of the fear that writing anything will turn out to be the confession of a crime. The Freudian discovery that behind the fear is the wish suggests that such a person is riddled with superego rigidity; the unconscious wish is to escape such superego pressure. The wish can therefore be to do something outrageously mischievous, or even illegal, in order to subvert such superego pressure. However, such a wish is so frightening that it is repressed. The result of the repression of such a wish forms the symptom of thinking of crime, correspondingly then feeling self-convicted, and then, of course, fearing punishment. Presumably, under it all is an original wish for the death of some influential early nuclear figure—a parent—and the difference between wishing and doing becomes rather nebulous in the person's psyche.

PSEUDOMNESIA The person believes something has taken place that, in fact, has never taken place. Analogous to hypnagogic hallucination with a dash of enosiophobia.

PSEUDONEUROTIC SCHIZOPHRENIA A diagnostic designation no longer utilized in the newer diagnostic nomenclatures. The chief symptom of this diagnosis is the characteristic presence of pan-anxiety; that is, anxiety that covers all spheres of the person's life. It is considered a basic psychotic underlay with a neurotic facade and, although erased as a modern conventional diagnosis, it remains, nevertheless, in a practical clinical sense useful with the pan-anxiety as the pathognomic sign of the diagnosis. Also referred to as micropsychosis.

PSEUDOQUERULANT A variant of the paranoid personality in which righteous indignation plays a central role in the person's constant vigilance regarding injustices. Such a disorder is usually seen as a lifelong characteristic of the personality.

PSI A parapsychological concept referring to a person's ostensible extrasensory ability.

PSYCHE Roughly equivalent to "mind," although also seen as an overarching conception of mind, where organization of cognitive as well as personality dynamics are governed.

PSYCHE, CONTRASEXUAL COMPONENT OF Jung's conception of the psyche as containing male and female components. The "soul image" of the man is the Anima, and of the woman the Animus. The theory holds that if these soul images are confused, then feminine qualities can appear in the male, and male qualities in the female.

PSYCHIATRIC NURSING A domain in the mental health field devoted to counseling care along with a wide variety of nursing concerns.

PSYCHIATRIC SOCIAL WORK Historically, a mental health discipline that applies mental health principles to casework practice. In contemporary mental health practice, psychiatric social workers are also psychotherapists and psychoanalysts and referred to as clinical social workers with the MSW or doctoral degree. In the past these professional social workers were mostly MSWs, although currently a greater number of doctoral-level social workers are seen.

PSYCHIATRIST A physician whose specialty is devoted to treatment of the mental disorders, either psychological, as in psychotherapy or with respect to other nonpsychological treatment such as pharmacological or electoconvulsive treatment.

PSYCHIATRY, FORENSIC The role of psychiatry in legal proceedings.

PSYCHIATRY, GERIATRIC The role of psychiatry in treating aging and elderly individuals.

PSYCHIC Of the psyche, as in the theoretical constructs psychic energy or psychic investment.

PSYCHICAL APPARATUS Freud's metapsychology can be defined as a discussion of the dynamics of mental states that can be illustrated by distinctions made between the unconscious, preconscious, and conscious, or between the ego, id, and superego, and how such dynamics operate. It is that aspect of the person that acts as an organizing metapsychology or abstraction that accounts for the relationship between phenomena of cognition, emotion, and motivation as well as other facets of the personality.

PSYCHIC PAIN A somatoform disorder defined as the condition of experiencing and complaining of pain in the face of negative physical findings. See Psychogenic pain disorder; Somatoform disorders.

PSYCHOACTIVE Referring to medications that are considered to be energizers.

PSYCHOACTIVE SUBSTANCE DEPENDENCE Referring to addiction to alcohol or to any variety of drugs.

PSYCHOANALYSIS A view of human development and behavior and a process of psychotherapy treatment based on the theory developed by Sigmund Freud. Guided by the principle of psychic determinism, the vicissitudes of the instincts along with early experiences are viewed as determining later psychological, behavioral, and symptomatic outcomes. Psychoanalysis includes salient concepts of the unconscious, repression, resistance, transference and its interpretation, wish fulfillment, intrapsychic conflict, symptom formation, dream interpretation, and psychosexual development, among a host of other metapsychological considerations covering the entire arena of psychopathology and development. A treatment technology is derived from these psychological and metapsychological concepts to address personality conflict and symptom formation. A major principle is that increased accessibility to consciousness is curative so that feelings need to be made conscious by overcoming defensive strategies erected against insight. Consciousness of repressed material and experiences presumably existing in a fragmentary state are invited into consciousness through dream and transference analysis and through the analysis of resistance. Psychoanalysis is considered to be a reconstructive psychotherapy so that the effects of instinctual drives, early psychosexual events of life, and overall irrational forces ultimately may be synthesized in a way that promotes reality testing over impulse, instinct, and overall irrationality. A small sample of the scores of contributors to the domain of psychoanalysis related to children as well as adults includes Abend, Arlow, Aron, Beres, Bergmann, H. Blum, Brenner, Bromberg, Eagle, Furst, Ganzarain, Gedo, Greenacre, Greenson, Greenspan, Grinstein, Lachmann, Lax, Lothane, Mitchell, Modell, Newirth, Ogden, Orgel, Pine, Rangell, Ritvo, Parens. Sandler, Stolorow, and Stone.

PSYCHOANALYSIS, META, AND DIAGNOSTICS A small sample of luminaries who, on the one hand, are responsible for theoretical contributions to the metapsychology of psychoanalysis and, on the other, to the psychoanalytic understanding of personality and diagnosis has included Merton Gill, Robert Holt, George Klein, Fred Pine, David Rapaport, Roy Schafer, and Robert Wallerstein.

PSYCHOANALYSIS, WILD The sort of psychotherapy characterized by invasive, confrontational approaches to the patient in a context of permeable therapist/patient boundaries.

PSYCHOANALYST Usually a clinical practitioner who holds a license in one of the four mental health licensed disciplines, which include clinical social worker, psychiatric nurse, psychiatrist, and psychologist. In addition, the psychoanalyst would also have been certificated from a bona fide psychoanalytic institute as a result of postgraduate training in psychoanalysis. In the most generic sense, a psychoanalyst is a psychodynamically oriented practitioner—including the relational therapist. In the specific sense, the psychoanalyst is a Freudian or neo-Freudian who is interested in relating a patient's historic material to present-day conflicts and, in so doing, analyzing transference, interpreting resistance, and penetrating repression.

PSYCHOBIOGRAPHY Also referred to as psychopathography. See Psychohistory.

PSYCHODIAGNOSTICS Referring to psychological tests used to gain an understanding of the personality and to facilitate the determination of a differential diagnosis. A sample of contributors to psychodiagnostic understanding include Lauretta Bender, Anthony Burry, John Exner, Robert Holt, Bruno Klopfer, Karen Machover, Fred Pine, David Rapaport, and Hermann Rorschach.

PSYCHODRAMA A form of psychotherapy that utilizes stage drama and role assignment to examine personal conflict and facilitate a more useful perspective for the person with respect to conflict and difficulties in relationships. See Moreno, J. L.

PSYCHODRAMATIC SHOCK A technique of Moreno's psychodrama in which the pathological trauma is reconstructed in order, ultimately, to implement controls over pathology.

PSYCHODYNAMICS The operation and interaction of the various forces of personality, including cognitive organization, emotional, psychological, and mental life, generally, and the effects of such phenomena, specifically.

PSYCHOGENIC Psychological, emotional, or particular mental problem that is not caused by an organic or biochemical disturbance, but rather by an emotional reaction to some encounter or by patterns of behavior based upon psychological motives.

PSYCHOGENIC AMNESIA A dissociative disorder in which there is a parsing of consciousness with respect to memory. See Dissociative disorders.

PSYCHOGENIC FUGUE A dissociative disorder in which there is a parsing of consciousness with respect to location. See Dissociative disorders.

PSYCHOGENIC MUTISM Psychologically caused loss of speech.

PSYCHOGENIC PAIN DISORDER A somatoform disorder resembling a physical disorder. See Somatoform disorders.

PSYCHOHISTORY Combining psychoanalytic and biographical data in order to further understand personality manifestations and to derive speculations of the person's psychology from implications of the data. Examples would be the many biographical investigations of Freud—notable among them Peter Gay's *Freud* or Paul Roazen's *The Trauma of Freud* as well as Irving Stone's biographical novel of Freud, *The Passion of the Mind*. Susan Kavaler-Adler's psychological investigations into the lives of women writers in her work *The Compulsion to Create* is also an example of psychobiography within the context of psychohistory.

PSYCHOIMMUNOLOGY The relation of immune system phenomena to psychological issues. The study of biological imperatives as they relate to possible emotional/psychological considerations.

PSYCHOLINGUISTICS The relation between language and psychology.

PSYCHOLOGICAL Pertaining to the study of behavior, emotions, mental functioning, and the overall approach to the relation between the higher mental functions and personality.

PSYCHOLOGICAL PILLOW A catatonia phenomenon in which the patient, while lying down, keeps the head raised just above the pillow.

PSYCHOLOGIST A licensed professional, with a doctoral degree in psychology (Ph.D. or Psy.D.), who is trained in scientific psychology and in any number of specialties including

cognitive behavior psychology—treating dysfunction with cognitive behavioral techniques in the here and now;

counseling psychology—focus on students and other counseling venues such as occupational;

developmental psychology—work with children and adolescents;

industrial psychology—commercial and industrial consultation;
neuropsychology—diagnosing neurological and organic brain disorders;
psychodynamic clinical psychology—therapy and diagnosis;
research and academic psychology—focus on psychological phenomena either by teaching and / or by laboratory work;
school psychology—employed in school systems to work with children, parents, and school personnel regarding student problems;
Social psychology—studying groups, their functions and effects.

There are other less well-known specialties:

anthropological psychology—cultural psychology. See Kardiner, Abraham;
comparative psychology—laboratory work with animals;
ethological psychology—study of animals in their natural environments.

PSYCHOMETRICS Psychologist's use of mental, psychological, emotional, intelligence, and vocational testing.

PSYCHOMOTOR Physical motion that is motivated psychologically and not organically.

PSYCHOMOTOR RETARDATION The slowing down of functioning (mental as well as physical), usually due to depression.

PSYCHONEUROSIS See Neurosis.

PSYCHONOETISM Reflecting a person's shift from emotional conflict to a specific focus on intellectual oppositionalism. Thus, rather than playing out the neurotic drama with respect to emotional conflict, the person plays it out intellectually so that ambivalence becomes a chief characteristic of the personality.

PSYCHOPATHIC PERSONALITY Generally considered an antisocial or sociopathic personality. Diagnostic factors include persistent acting out, repression of anger, absence of anxiety, shame, or guilt, an ostensible fear of what is clinically considered a silent inner life (requiring endless external stimulation). Considered a psychogenic disorder based upon childhood neglect and abuse, also reflecting a contaminated superego, or the harboring of paranoid impulses to hurt another in order to prevent being hurt by that other. Referred to in modern *DSM* nosology as an Axis II personality disorder called antisocial personality disorder. See Personality / character disorder.

PSYCHOPATHOLOGY The phenomenon of disorders of mental, emotional, psychological, and cognitive dynamics. It is likely that inherent in all psychopathology is the emotion and effect of anger on the personality. A small sample of contributors of this domain include Agras, Akiskal, Andreason, Arieti, Burry, Clayton, Cloninger, Costello, Kellerman, Kernberg, and Klerman. See Anger; Symptoms.

PSYCHOPHARMACOLOGY The use of medication in the treatment of psychological, emotional, and organic disorders. A sample of psychiatrists known for expertise in the general arena of psychopharmacological treatment include Robert Cancro, Ronald Fieve, Donald F. Klein, and Andrew Slaby.

PSYCHOPHYSIOLOGIC DISORDERS Synonymous with psychosomatic or somatization disorders; that is, physical manifestations thought to be caused by emotional and psychological forces. Emphasized by Franz Alexander.

PSYCHOSEXUAL Either referring to sexual disorders or a reference to psychosexual stages of development construed by Freud to include the oral, anal, phallic, and oedipal phases of development—from birth through ages four or five—along with the stage of latency till adolescence. See Freud, Sigmund.

PSYCHOSIS Essentially a disorder of failed reality testing, including hallucinations, delusions, and / or mood pathology, and manifested in the schizophrenias, the affective pathologies, as well as in organic brain syndromes.

PSYCHOSIS, FURLOUGH A psychotic so-called break seen among soldiers who arrive home from active duty. Some such individuals experience symptoms presumably as a result of either a delayed reaction to the stress of military life or to the absence of the rules, regulations, and structure of military life.

PSYCHOSIS, MALIGNANT The type of psychosis that continues to worsen into an extreme dementia.

PSYCHOSIS, MANIC-DEPRESSIVE An example of the affective psychoses. This affective psychosis can appear as a manic condition, a depressive condition, or as a serial manic and then depressive cycle. In the manic state, the person is exceedingly energized (super expressed), and in the depressive state, the person is exceedingly withdrawn, inert, and depressed (not expressed). Referred to in *DSM* nosology in the category of mood disorders. See Bipolar disorder; Depression, *DSM* diagnoses.

PSYCHOSIS, REACTIVE Analagous to reactive depression insofar as the psychosis is a response to a situational event. It is designed to evade the emotional turmoil of the event, just as in reactive depression (of prior *DSM* nosology) the depression is an attempt to allay the anxiety of a recent traumatic event.

PSYCHOSIS, SCHIZOAFFECTIVE A type of schizophrenia referred to in *DSM* nomenclature as a schizoaffective psychosis in which the affective dysfunction, such as a major manic or major depressive episode, is so severe that it masks the schizophrenic structure of the basic dynamic.

PSYCHOSIS, SCHIZOPHRENIFORM A form of reactive psychosis with a decent prognosis, especially with relatively normal premorbid activity.

PSYCHOSIS, SYMBIOTIC INFANTILE Mahler's concept regarding a panic state during the infant's separation from mother, resulting in the child's projection of the tension-rage and then, of course, seeing hostility from the world. The solution is that the child may regress to an omnipotent position. Hallucinations and / or delusions may be present.

PSYCHOSIS, TRAUMATIC Caused by any number of brain injuries.

PSYCHOSOCIAL EFFECTS Environmental / cultural elements that affect psychological functioning.

PSYCHOSOMATIC DISORDERS See psychophysiologic disorders.

PSYCHOSURGERY Brain surgery designed to modify emotions. Historically, frontal lobe surgery was designed to nullify rage reactions as well as other cognitive maladaptions. Unfortunately, patients were then frequently found in a vegetative state, typically sitting and staring, in the absence of any normal emotional color. Prefrontal lobotomies were performed from 1935 into about the mid twentieth century.

PSYCHOSYNTHESIS Introduced by the Italian psychiatrist Roberto Assagioli (1888–1974). The psyche is a tripartite system:

the lower unconscious—the person's past;
the middle unconscious—things that can be brought into consciousness;
the superconscious—creativity and sense of heroic action exist.

The aim of psychosynthesis therapy is to continue, in a series of successive approximations, to create ever higher or greater syntheses between these parts, at the same time decreasing any conflict among these functions. Therapeutic techniques include those that will better coordinate and reorganize the person's attitudes and values, so that these greater syntheses can be achieved. Influences include Jung and Maslow.

PSYCHOTHERAPIST A designation of a person practicing talk therapy in the absence of any specific license that would correspond to a particular mental health discipline.

PSYCHOTHERAPY Any system with a number of directed interventions that is based upon corresponding theoretical underpinnings in order to impact personality in a way that claims to alter self-defeating behaviors as well as assuage, reduce, or otherwise treat psychopathology. Supportive and/or brief psychotherapy aims to strengthen ego by reviewing the patient's behavior and, through various methods, reduce tension. Behavior and cognitive behavior therapies aim to erase conditioned responses through behavioral reconditioning and cognitive shifts, the result of using various behavioral/cognitive techniques. Psychodynamic psychotherapies aim to engage a process of deepening psychodynamic understanding by working with psychological tools of transference interpretation, analysis of the patient's resistance, and the tracing of defense mechanisms. A small sample of clinicians reflecting the range of approaches from directive, confrontational modalites to nondirective approaches include Charles Brenner, Abraham I. Cohen, Darlene Ehrenberg, Albert Ellis, Priscilla Kauff, Steven Knoblauch, Robert Langs, Robert Marshall, Simone Marshall, Fritz Perls, Carl Rogers, Paul Wachtel, and Lewis Wolberg. The scope of specific therapies and their underpinnings include Freudian to Gestalt, Jungian to Morita, cognitive behavior to psychodrama, Rogerian client centered to paradoxical, Adlerian to Sullivanian, Kleinian to Horneyan, transactional to transpersonal, Yoga to psychosynthesis, Naikan therapy to ego psychology and the relational therapies, rational emotive behavior therapy to object relations formulations, and intersubjective understanding to confrontational approaches.

PSYCHOTHERAPY INSTITUTES A sample of such institutes includes Albert Ellis Institute (NY), Atlanta Center for Cognitive Therapy, Baltimore Washington Society and Institute, C. G. Jung Institute of San Francisco, C. G. Jung Institute of Chicago, Center for Cognitive Therapy (Oakland, California), Center for Dialectical and Cognitive Behavioral Therapies (Long Island, NY), Cognitive Behavioral Institute of Albuquerque, Center for Modern Psychoanalytic Studies (Boston), Dallas Psychoanalytic Institute, Denver Institute for Psychoanalysis, Freeman International Institute for Cognitive Therapy (Fort Wayne), Gestalt Center for Psychotherapy and Training (NY), Gestalt Center for Gainesville, Gestalt Therapy Institute of Los Angeles, Gestalt Therapy Institute of Philadelphia, Gestalt Institute of Austin, Gestalt Institute of San Francisco, Institute of Contemporary Psychotherapy (Los Angeles), Institute for the Psychoanalytic Study of Subjectivity (NY), Manhattan Institute of Psychoanalysis, National Institute of the Psychotherapies (NY), National Psychological Association for Psychoanalysis (NY), New Center for Psychoanalysis (Los Angeles), New York C. G. Jung Institute, New York Institute for Gestalt Therapy, New York Psychoanalytic Institute, Object Relations Institute for Psychotherapy and Psychoanalysis (NY), Pacific Gestalt Institute (Los Angeles), Postgraduate Center for Mental Health (NY), Washington Center for Psychoanalysis, Training Institute for Mental Health (NY), San Francisco Center for Psychoanalysis, Training Institute for Mental Health (NY), Washington Center for Psychoanalysis (NY), Washington Square Institute for Psychotherapy (NY), William Alanson White Institute (NY).

PSYCHOTHERAPY VECTORS The therapist's understanding or empathy toward the patient is not a panacea for cure. The absolutely strongest force is the patient's pathology that will not in the slightest be affected by any sole empathy or even by complete dissolution of resistance. Thus pathology is considered the strongest of the vectors that influence treatment effectiveness. It is hypothesized that addressing pathology requires at least a mandatory raising of the consciousness (out of repression) of anger toward some targeted object in order for anything resembling cure to be claimed. Thus, Freud's proposition that consciousness is curative is an important step in clarifying how pathology can be penetrated. The only qualifier to this proposition concerns the core issue of what exactly it is that needs to be made conscious in order for powerful therapeutic effects to address psychopathology. When the repressed anger toward a significant object (concealed in the unconscious) is surfaced, then, and perhaps only then, can the pathology be addressed. The question whether there is anything stronger than the patient's pathology is now also possibly addressed: Yes, consciousness is powerfully curative, provided that what becomes conscious is the patient's anger toward another (the object), which was hitherto repressed. The associated axiom would be: No subject matter, other than unrepressing the anger toward the object, can be curative. See Therapeutic vectors.

PSYCHOTIC See psychosis.

PSYCHOTOMIMETIC Mimicking psychosis as a function of the ingestion of a drug.

PSYCHOTROPIC DRUGS Medicinal agents used to control dynsfunctional or abberant mental/emotional/psychological conditions. There are several such categories of psychotropic drugs:

antidepressants—energizers;
antimanic agents—lithium;
anxiolytic sedatives—tranquilizers and anti-anxiety agents;
neuroleptics—antipsychotics;
psychostimulants—amphetamines;
psychodysleptics—psychedelics.

PUBERTY Roughly the beginning of the adolescent phase of life with the appearance of secondary sex characteristics. Psychoanalytically, it is proposed that this phase ushers in the reexperiencing, in a much more latent form, the oral, anal, and phallic cathexes of the prelatency phase.

PUBESCENCE Puberty.

PUERILISM The stage after infancy.

PUNITIVE STRUCTURE An anger, or denoting blame psychology, and borrowed from social psychology. There are three parts to blame psychology—including one of nonblame as a contrasting condition:

intrapunitive—blaming the self;
extrapunitive—blaming the object (others);
impunitive—nonblame condition; implies a striving for objectivity in the absence of anger or blame.

PYKNIC TYPE See Sheldon, William Herbert.

PYROMANIA Fire-setting inclination.

Q

Q-SORT A multidimensional rating technique used in the evaluation of personality traits and attitudes, assessed through the comparison of several raters.

QUALITY, DETERMINING Identifying the historical pivotal event in hysterical diagnosis, which reveals the power of the original trauma. Conceived by Freud.

QUATERNITY Referring to the amalgam of four factors as might be applied to Jungian theory with respect to archetypes. The number 4 was important in Jung's formulations. See Jung, Carl Gustav.

QUERULENT A trait of personality that is given easily to anger and demonstrates righteous indignation, oppositionalism, protest, dissatisfaction. See Pseudoquerulent.

QUOTIENT, INTELLIGENCE See Intelligence Quotient.

R

RACHMAN, ARNOLD W. (1936–). American psychologist/psycholanalyst. Instrumental in energizing the renaissance of interest in the history and the work of Sandor Ferenczi. Scholar of the history of psychoanalysis. A sample of other scholars of Ferenczi include Aron, Brabant, Dupont, Gedo, Haynal, Thompson, and Wolstein. See Ferenczi, Sandor.

RADO, SANDOR (1890–1972). European-born American psychiatrist. Promoted adaptational psychoanalysis and studied sexual orientation. Also promoted the use of aversion therapy—negative thoughts are forcibly negatively associated in order to unlearn homosexual impulse and behavior.

RAGE Intense anger, fury.

RAGE, DEFIANT Related to protest behavior. Rado coined this phrase to indicate the particular defiance toward authority that is first seen during the terrible twos.

RAGE, SHAM Organic disorder first seen in animals and reflecting sudden expostulations of rage in humans. It is a laboratory-induced rage.

RANK, OTTO (1884–1939). European psychoanalyst best known for his birth trauma theory, in which all pathology can be ultimately traced to the trauma of being born. Developed a theory of will. Will therapy is essentially the struggle an individual can invite to seek autonomy rather than remain in a dependent condition. The person can defeat neurosis by force of will. Differed from Freud insofar as Rank considered a focus on the past a distraction or defense against feeling things in the present.

RAPAPORT, DAVID (1911–1960). European-born American psychologist influential in the conceptualization of the metapsychology of psychoanalysis. Clarified the nature of ego functions and, with Gill and Schafer, worked on a psychodiagnostic assessment from an ego psychology theoretical viewpoint.

RAPE FANTASY Seen in both males and females, although claimed to be more frequently fantasized by female individuals who are in positions of power. Rape fantasies also exist in cases where the person shows a passive inclination. In terms of psychoanalytic understanding, it may be hypothesized that, where the superego is severe (and even tyrannical), erotic excitation may be wrenched from the psyche's superego control and is therefore expressed by the subject without the psyche (the subject) holding its conscious self responsible. Thus, with respect to the superego, the rape fantasy accomplishes the aim of achieving sexual freedom (climax) by virtue of the subject's capitulation to the libido.

RAPID EYE MOVEMENT See REM (Rapid Eye Movement).

RAPPORT The key to establishing a good working relationship in the therapeutic endeavor. Rapport is the consolidation of reciprocity of empathy and trust. It involves the all-important element of "feeling understood." A case could be made that rapport is the most important factor in the therapeutic process, although, with respect to the concept of resistance, not solely in a positive way, and despite protestations to the contrary, the achievement of rapport certainly cannot address and penetrate psychopathology on its own. See Therapeutic vectors.

RAPPROCHEMENT Mahler's object relations concept. From sixteen months to two years of life the child tries to manage a more independent stance beyond a symbiotic connection to mother.

RAPTUS Associated with catatonic schizophrenia, where the sufferer will suddenly react with motor behavior. Seen as an attempt to lessen tension. See Schizophrenia.

RATIONAL EMOTIVE BEHAVIOR THERAPY (REBT) The first of the cognitive behavior therapies, REBT (originally called rational therapy) was developed in 1955 by American psychologist Albert Ellis as an alternative to psychoanalysis. REBT is a comprehensive approach to psychological problems that emphasizes the interrelationship of cognition, emotion, and behavior. It is posited on the notion that self-defeating beliefs or schemas, acquired in early childhood, are perpetuated through a continued process of self-reindoctrination. REBT teaches people how to control their own emotional destiny by identifying maladaptive, illogical, and self-defeating beliefs, then forcefully challenging them and replacing them with more rational and adaptive thoughts and behaviors. Major focus in REBT is on unconditional acceptance of self and others and toleration of difficult life circumstances. The goal here is to decrease dysfunctional emotions such as depression, anxiety, or anger and replace them with the more adaptive ones of disappointment, regret, or concern, thus facilitating other changes, such as more effective problem solving and relational skills. REBT's applications have extended into areas such as education, business, social change and philosophy. See ABCDE; Ellis, Albert.

RATIONALIZATION In psychoanalytic understanding, rationalization is usually an unconscious defensive attempt to adjust thinking in order to justify one's motivation and behavior. Considered an ego defense and often used by people with obsessional disorders in conjunction with the defense style of intellectualization. See Defense mechanisms.

RAT MAN A seminal case presented by Freud of a man who was gripped with the obsessional idea of rats in an overturned bowl cannibalizing a person by boring into the anus. This was a torture that the Rat Man, while serving in the military, had heard was typical in the Far East. The subject experienced dread and was obsessed by the fear that it could happen to him or even to his father and fiancée. Freud saw the obsession as a neurosis in which the conflict was between loving and aggressive impulses and also interpreted the fantasy as masking homosexual fantasies.

RBs (RATIONAL BELIEFs) See ABCDE.

REACTION FORMATION An ego defense originally implying the demonstration of an opposite emotional reaction to an original feeling. Thus, excessive sweetness can be used to mask an aggressive desire to dominate and suffocate, as in "killing with kindness." Refined by Kellerman to mean an aversive opposite reaction to any stimulus that is attractive to the subject (such as a forbidden pleasure) as dictated by a superego judgment. For example, in dreams, a reaction of revulsion to the sight of a family member in some state of undress would be considered, from a psychoanalytic oedipal point of view, the reaction to a basic attraction. The basic attraction is considered to be unacceptable. Hence the substitute reaction of revulsion is designed to head off consciousness of the presumed instant impulse of attraction. The original definition of reaction formation has essentially been replaced by the defense known as turning into the opposite. Reaction formation is applicable in a number of diagnostic syndromes, but especially in obsessive and manic personalities. See Defense mechanisms; Opposite, reversal into the.

REACTION TIME In all sorts of psychological and cognitive tests, a typical measure of the subject's time lag between the presentation of the stimulus and the subject's response to the stimulus.

REACTIVE DEPRESSION See Depression, reactive.

REALITY PRINCIPLE One of two principles proposed by Freud to explain the governance of mental activity. The reality principle is a learned one and is a function of development. In contrast, the pleasure principle is innate. The reality principle aids in instinctual gratification by promoting understanding and action according to external demands, while the pleasure principle leads to relief of instinctual tension through the venues of wish fulfillment. See Pleasure-pain principle.

REALITY TESTING Observing and understanding the external world and responding in a way that faithfully reflects the realistic requirements of such external conditions.

REBT (RATIONAL EMOTIVE BEHAVIOR THERAPY) Albert Ellis's formulation of the ABCDE of this approach to psychotherapy. See ABCDE; Ellis, Albert; Rational emotive behavior therapy (REBT).

RECIDIVISM Repetition of delinquent or criminal activity.

RECIPROCAL INHIBITION Behavior therapy counterconditioning technique, introduced by South African–born American psychiatrist Joseph Wolpe, aimed at replacing an undesired response with a more adaptive one that neutralizes the anxiety potentiated by the stimulus. See Counterconditioning; Systematic desensitization.

RECONSTRUCTIVE PSYCHOTHERAPY Referring to psychodynamic / psychoanalytic approaches that aim to create corrective behavior through the working through of historic conflicts as these manifest themselves through the transference to the analyst.

REDUCTIONISM A philosophical position proposing that a nomological network or theoretical system can be reduced to basic elements. Psychoanalysis is an example of a reductionist underpinning.

REFERENTIAL INTEGRATION An emotional informational processing perspective related to the implicit relational knowing of intersubjectivity theory.

REFRAMING In REBT and cognitive behavior therapy, this is relabeling behavior by putting it into a new, more positive perspective. In family therapy, reframing refers to cognitive restructuring of the family dynamic with respect to developing different views of existing symptoms of the family. See Family therapy; Rational emotive behavior therapy.

REFRIGERATOR PARENTS Parents who are emotionally cold and who were, in the past, mistakenly thought to be responsible for the autism of children.

REGRESSION An ego defense that enables the subject to recede to previous levels of functioning. Also seen in subjects who act out, and, in this sense, regression is a typical defense of the psychopathic (antisocial) diagnostic type. In severe regression, schizophrenia becomes an obvious diagnosis. See Defense mechanisms.

REGRESSION IN THE SERVICE OF THE EGO A psychoanalytic precept regarding the operation of regression within the process of free association. The stream of consciousness during free association can create a loosening of superego controls, but, because of the patient's ego strength, this uncovering or recession (regression) becomes a creative pursuit (sans superego control) of historic material (feelings toward other historic figures) in service of the treatment. The patient then regains ego traction to reconstitute basic ego reality structure.

REICH, WILHELM (1897–1957). European-born American psychiatrist/psychoanalyst. Best known for his orgone box (designed to cure sexual incapacity). Reich claimed that this discovery, orgone, was an energy that permeated all matter. His focus on orgone body work ultimately influenced body-oriented therapies as well as Gestalt, and primal therapy. However, his main contribution to theoretical dynamic psychopathology was in the unfolding of the origin, inner workings, and development of character structure.

REIFICATION Synonymous with concretization.

REIK, THEODOR (1888–1969). European-born American psychologist. One of Freud's first students and reputed to have written the first psychoanalytic Ph.D. dissertation. Prolific author best known for his books *The Compulsion to Confess, Masochism and Modern Man, Listening with the Third Ear, The Secret Self,* and *Myth and Guilt.* His published works include analyses of masochism, guilt, love, self-analysis, and the unconscious. In certain respects he is a progenitor of Lacanian psychology, intersubjective investigation, as well as influencing the study of countertransference. Founded the National Psychological Association for Psychoanalysis, a psychoanalytic institute that included students and faculty who, over the decades, have become significant contributors to the theory and practice of psychotherapy. These include Lawrence Balter, Martin S. Bergmann, Reuben Fine, Harold Greenwald, Emanuel Hammer, Althea Horner, Robert Lindner, Nancy McWilliams, and Robert D. Stolorow.

REINFORCEMENT Increasing the frequency or probability of a response by presentation of a reward or removal of an aversive stimulus following a response.

Positive reinforcement—process of increasing the probability of a desired reaction to a stimulus through rewarding the behavior when it occurs.

Negative reinforcement—process of reducing the probability of an undesired response to a stimulus by following the undesired response with an aversive stimulus.

RELABELING A family therapy concept regarding roles. See Reframing.

RELATIONAL PSYCHOTHERAPY Relationship between patient and analyst is mutually constituted so that the therapist is not a blank screen (as in classical psychoanalysis); that is, both analyst and patient understand the objective world through a shared subjectivity. Analogous to quantum theory, whereby that which is measured is affected by the act of measurement. Bridges the theories of object relations, interpersonal psychotherapy, and intersubjective psychology. A major influence on the view of relational psychotherapy is the contemporary psychologist/psychoanalyst Stephen A. Mitchell. See Mitchell, Stephen A.

REM (RAPID EYE MOVEMENT) This phase of sleep is associated with increased physiologic activity as well as the presence of dreaming.

REM BEHAVIOR DISORDER (RBD) A parasomnia (sleep disruption) in which the sleeper will have disturbed dreams along with violent behavior during REM (dream) sleep. See Parasomnia.

REMISSION "The person is in remission" is the phrase used by clinicians to indicate that whatever disturbance was present is no longer in effect. This improvement and the receding of the disturbance is thought to be one in which the disturbance is held in abeyance, but not necessarily in a state of permanent cure; the disturbance may also be in partial remission.

REMORSE Feeling of regret, but not necessarily of guilt.

RENUNCIATION, INSTINCTUAL In psychoanalytic understanding, renouncing an instinct is translated into the ego saying "No" to the id. This is so, because not to renounce the instinct is presumably to place the subject (or ego) in danger.

REPARATION When, as a result of guilt or rage, an object in fantasy has been practically destroyed, the reparative process in psychotherapy is a result of a reinvestigation and reconfiguring of the conflict so that the patient is able to treat the problem more maturely. The reparative process addresses the patient's ambivalence.

REPETITION COMPULSION This Freudian insight reveals that a person will (obsessively and compulsively) repeat some behavior as a way of trying to master an original anxiety. Of course, doing that in the here and now can have no real affect on the original problem. The repetition continues to reinforce a repression of a memory.

REPRESSED, RETURN OF THE Involuntary surfacing into consciousness of previously held material from the unconscious.

REPRESSION The chief ego defense mechanism that keeps unacceptable impulses out of consciousness. Facets of repression exist in all defenses. Other perspectives on repression consider concepts such as

1. perceptual defense (you don't see what you don't want to see);
2. failure to make meaningful connections (not seeing key relationships);
3. failure to formulate the unformulated (known thoughts, unknown);
4. unable to understand inner stimuli (not crystallizing intuition);
5. focusing exclusively on positive illusions (avoiding a consistent focus on external reality signals);

6. typical use of denial mechanisms (equivalent to selective perception—seeing only what you want to see); and
7. reliance on an attachment pattern that is avoidant and dismissive (keeping one in a behind the line position), along with the use of characteristic avoidant defenses.

In psychodynamic psychology, repression is among a select few psychological phenomena occupying a major role in all of psychopathology. See Defense mechanisms; Unconscious.

RESEARCH DIAGNOSTIC CRITERIA (RDC) A clinical profile that lists those symptoms that are pathognomonic of schizophrenia. See Pathognomonic.

RESIDUAL SCHIZOPHRENIA See Schizophrenia.

RESIDUE, NIGHT Leftover material from the previous night, as in the recall of a dream.

RESIGNATION, NEUROTIC A concept developed by Karen Horney to denote one of the person's strategies and tactics to avoid conflict and evade confrontation with stimuli that are personally noxious or upsetting or represent the assumption of a dependent position.

RESISTANCE A central concept in the psychoanalytic process reflecting the person's unconscious striving to keep conflictual material repressed. Therefore, the main purpose of resistance in treatment is to support repression and therefore, maintain symptoms. Psychoanalysts see the patient's rejection of all interpretation as a function of the patient's resistance. Therapists then target the overcoming of such resistances as the major curative tactic, especially when the resistance appears as a transference resistance.

Ego resistance—equivalent to general resistance and its support of repression.

Id resistance—arguably the strongest resistance insofar as it relies on the use of the repetition-compulsion and becomes the last bastion of defense once the state of the ego resistance is weakened.

Superego resistance—resistance of the therapy based upon the patient's guilt and masochism, which supports a permeating negative transference as a defense against an expectation that the therapist will withdraw love.

See Transference resistance.

RESTITUTION In schizophrenia, this is the person's attempt to regain a hold on reality (restitution) as a result of the massive regression that presumably had taken place.

RESTRICTORS Referring to anorexia, where food intake is severely impoverished, in contrast to other eating disorders such as bulimia in which the person will eat and intermittently gorge.

RETARDATION See Mental retardation.

RETRANSCRIBING ACTION OF THE HIPPOCAMPUS In the domain of neuropsychoanalysis, repression is a function of hormones that shut off the retranscribing action of the hippocampus. Schore suggests that repression represents left brain cognitive inhibition of right brain affective processes. See Repression.

RETROGRADE, AMNESIA See Amnesia.

RETT'S DISORDER A deceleration of head growth seen in the child between the ages of five and forty-eight months. Along with this, there is a loss of hand skills, poor gait and coordination, poor motor behavior, and impaired language development. See Pervasive developmental disorders.

REVERIE Drifting in daydreams.

REVERSAL See Opposite, reversal into the.

RIGHT BRAIN EMOTIONAL PROCESSES According to Schore, in the domain of neuropsychoanalysis, the early developing right brain correlates to processing and regulation of affects at all points in the lifespan in all intimate contexts—including the therapeutic alliance—and further, has implications for the infrastructure of psychopathology.

ROAZEN, PAUL (1936–2005). American political scientist whose intellectual life was devoted to scholarly investigations into psychoanalytic theory. Published works on Freud and the psychoanalytic movement.

ROGERS, CARL (1902–1987). American psychologist who developed a model of "humanistic" psychotherapy in which the patient is referred to as a client, and the issue of accurate empathy in addition to an accurate focus on the client's needs form cornerstones of the approach. With respect to the technique of the therapist, and in order to achieve the best possible rapport in the therapy, reflection of the client's feelings rather than problem solving becomes the therapeutic objective. Rogerian proponents view their psychotherapy, theorized as the "actualizing tendency," to be client centered, and, along with Maslow, generating a philosophy. In terms of the issue of needs, Rogers proposed several components:

Organismic valuing—we know automatically what is good.
Positive regard—love and nurturance is natural.
Positive self-regard—we learn this by feedback from others.
Conditions of worth—we get things in a trade-off by being good.
Conditional positive regard—we bend to the wishes of others.
Conditional positive self-regard—we like ourselves if we meet standards that are given to us by others.
Real self—when all good things happen, then one can be the real self.
Ideal self—living by standards set by others.
Incongruity—the gap between the real self and the ideal self: I am, versus I should.

To be a fully functioning person involves the following:

Openness to experience—opposite of defensiveness.
Existential living—living in the here and now.
Organismic trusting—should trust ourselves.
Experiential freedom—take responsibility for choices we make.
Creativity—giving back to others.

Further, in this client-centered therapy Rogers proposes that the therapist needs to have an "unconditional personal regard" for the client, and this refers to a core element that leads to development of healthier responses in the client. Along with unconditional personal regard, the therapist needs to have empathy for the client to better appreciate the client's inner world. Third, "genuineness," "transparency," or "congruence," is the therapist's awareness of feelings about the client, of which the therapist needs to be aware.

ROLE CONFUSION Equivalent to identity confusion.

ROLE-PLAY Technique used in cognitive behavior therapy to help clients rehearse different behaviors and cognitions in preparation for handling stressful situations or interactions.

Rational role reversal—an REBT technique in which the therapist voices aloud the client's irrational beliefs and the client vigorously counters them with rational statements.

ROLE REVERSAL Usually seen in families where one member inappropriately assumes the role of another member—especially if the new role exceeds the ability of the one assuming the role.

ROLFE, IDA PAULINE (1896–1979). American biochemist who developed technique called structural integration. See Rolfing.

ROLFING Soft tissue massage or manipulation with the assumption that psychic energies will be released in the service of healing. In this system, muscle is considered to have memory. The massage is designed to work on tissue in order to break down tension. Rolfe influenced the development of a number of body-oriented therapies and deep-massage systems as well as Gestalt therapy. Rolfe believed in organizing human structure in conformity with gravity.

RORSCHACH TEST Projective test developed by Hermann Rorschach, a Swiss psychiatrist (1884–1922). Responses to the ten ink blots are purported to reveal the inner dynamic psychic organization, character structure, and diagnosis of the subject. Concepts of the Rorschach include

Location of Percepts: Where Did You See It?

- *W*—a percept that refers to the entire ink blot insofar as the subject sees the entire blot as the particular object itself, rather than seeing only a detail, or part of the blot as an object. A reasonable number of *W*s indicate decent organizational ability, while a preponderance of such responses can suggest a passive orientation in the subject.
- *DW*—use of a large detail of the blot to explain the entire blot. It is understood to be a confabulated response meaning that it is likely produced by a person who is compelled more by an inner signal than by conventional reality signals. Considered to be an indication of pathology.
- *D*—refers to a large detail of the ink blot the subject chooses as defining a percept. A reasonable frequency of *D*s can be considered to reflect the person's ability to implement activity to reach a goal, rather than only thinking about a goal, but not doing much about it.
- *Dd*—location of a lesser-sized percept within a decent-sized larger detail of the blot. It is considered a facet of balance in the personality when, to a reasonable extent, such percepts are represented in the scoring profile of the test.
- *d*—located by the subject in a smaller detail of the whole ink blot. A rather large frequency of such responses can imply an obsessive characterological approach.
- *dd*—a preponderance of tiny detail responses reflects an obsessional and perhaps even overpersonalized, idiosyncratic ideation.
- *de*—edge detail (*de*) location of percepts reflect highly idiosyncratic ideation to the extent of being considered guarded or characterologically paranoid. It is the kind of response location that resembles a penumbra of the ink blot—a figurative shadowy edge—but not in the sense of the blot's texture.
- *S*—the use of the space as foreground instead of background, and a sufficient number of such reversals

presumably indicates an oppositional attitude in the personality.

Determinants: What Influenced Seeing It?

- *F*—the scoring of percepts that the subject selects based upon the form of the blot. High scores of *F* reflect a focus on the personality's needs for control.
- *M*—a human movement response. A preponderance of such responses, especially when the form of the percept is well articulated, is said to correlate with high intelligence and maturity level. Diagnostically and proportionally, such responses correspond more to the control obsessional side, in contrast to impulse on the hysterical side.
- *FM*—an animal movement response, meaning that the subject sees the form of an animal in motion in the ink blot. A preponderance of such responses, along with a paucity of the *M* response (human movement), suggests a more immature level of functioning.
- *Fc*—reflects control over tensions insofar as the *c* is a purported measure of anxiety or tension, while the *F* implies control. This *c* is the determinant for shading responses.
- *cF*—implies that the person's level of tension may be prevailing over control efforts in the personality.
- *c*—if the shading is the predominant reason for seeing the percept of the blot, then it is considered that, as this score accumulates, anxiety interferes to large measure in the personality.
- *F–F* minus scores on the Rorschach will be interpreted as reflecting a psychotic condition. The *F* minus is seen as a strong sign of poor reality testing, akin to the appearance of prevailing transparencies on the Machover Draw a Person Test.
- *FC*—when the determination of the percept is primarily animated by the form, and only secondarily by the color (*FC*), then a stronger picture of the ego begins to emerge, because the form element of perception is correlated with control over impulse.

- *CF*—when color dominates form (*CF*), controls are presumably less well developed, although these controls are better represented than responses determined only by pure color (*C*).
- *C*—the determinant for color, purported to measure the extent of emotional expressiveness. When the reason for seeing a particular percept on the test is solely determined by the color (*C*), it is said the person is dominated by impulse.

Some Result References

- *O*—Original response. The original response is different from the popular response insofar as it is a response to the blot that is infrequently given by subjects: correlated to creativity and high intelligence.
- *R*—the sum of all the responses, signaling an indirect general sense of the richness of the personality, qualified by any preponderance of responses indicating extreme obsessional, impulsive, poor reality testing responses (*F-*) or any other particular loading of pathological responses.
- *Affect ratio*—this is the ratio of responses of chromatic to achromatic cards, indicating the extent to which the subject can access emotion.

R PREFRONTAL CORTEX See Brain, emotional.

RUMINATE Obsessional thinking accompanied by withdrawal and compensatory fantasy. It is a persistent focus on an issue and, more often than not, reflects the subject's tension concerns.

S

SABOTEUR, INTERNAL See Internal saboteur.

SADISM Named after Marquis de Sade (1740–1814), the French writer whose observations revealed that sexual pleasure and/or orgasm for certain individuals is achieved when inflicting pain and/or humiliation on the partner. In the psychiatric *DSM* nomenclature, sexual sadism is referred to as a paraphilia. Psychoanalytically, sadism is considered to be an acting out of anal phase and phallic castration fears through their reversal—the devaluation, punishment, or humiliation of others. In addition, the disempowerment of the other (especially in sadism's extreme form) is understood as a compensatory elevation of the sadist's empowerment. This compensatory elevation permits a projective identification to occur, so that the sadist can identify with the disempowerment (as a vicarious experience), albeit in the absence of any sense of castration or devaluation or any derivative experience of disempowerment. Usually sadistic individuals are also more than just casually interested in forms of violence. See Paraphilia

SADOMASOCHISM The coexistence of both sadistic as well as masochistic impulses. In interpersonal relationships, the sadomasochistic interaction is performed by both partners in tandem; one assumes the role of the sadist, the other of the masochist. To satisfy the clinical condition of sadomasochism, the elements of sadism and masochism must be far more intense than mere aggression and passivity. It is also possible for the sadomasochistic partners to switch roles.

SAHS-UAO An acronym for sleep apnea hypersomnolence syndrome, which is concomitant with what is known as upper airway obstruction (UAO). Listed within the category of sleep disorders. See Sleep apnea.

SANGUINE Derived from one of the four humors of the early Greek physician Hippocrates. See Hippocrates.

SCAPEGOAT Anger, hostility, and aggression toward others as a projection of one's own fears and insecurities. An aspect of blame psychology.

SCATOLOGY Obsession with filth and excrement along with derivative behavior such as lewd phone calls.

SCATTERED SPEECH Typical in hebephrenic schizophrenia, indicating incoherence.

SCHACHTER, STANLEY (1922–). American psychologist who along with Singer developed the cognitive arousal theory, which postulates that a stimulus causes physiological arousal that is perceived to be an emotional state. Along with this, it is considered that emotional reactions are determined by an individual's interpretation of a situation.

SCHAFER, ROY (1922–). American psychoanalyst. Shifted from typical Freudian concepts of energy and drive to the position that to understand reality one must follow rules of language. Therefore, communicative psychology becomes more valuable than psychoanalytic metapsychology (with its foundations in the natural sciences of physics and biology).

SCHEDULE OF AFFECTIVE DISORDERS AND SCHIZOPHRENIA (SADS) An instrument that utilizes the data from the Research Diagnostic Criteria (RDC) to establish a definitive diagnosis.

SCHEMA Core dysfunctional beliefs systems about oneself, others, or the world, acquired in childhood when needs were not met, which serve as filters for our adult experiences. Common schemas include "I'm profoundly defective and unlovable;" "The world is a dangerous place;" and "Strong emotions must be suppressed." Useful in cognitive behavioral treatment as a means of assessing areas to be focused on that usually operate out of our awareness but, when triggered by an event, influence our cognitions, emotions and behavior. See Schema therapy; Young, Jeffrey E.

SCHEMA MODE In schema therapy, the three maladaptive coping styles through which schemas exert their influence: schema surrender, avoidance, and overcompensation.

SCHEMA THERAPY An outgrowth of cognitive behavior therapy developed by American psychologist Jeffrey Young. Especially useful in treating personality disorders utilizing long-held deeper cognitive structures as a means of treating problem moods and behaviors. Requires detailed history in combination with Young's Schema Questionnaire in order to distill client's core beliefs; employs cognitive therapy, experiential, Gestalt, and interpersonal therapy techniques and attachment and object relations theory. Ultimate goal is to fortify a person's healthy side by systematically confronting and challenging maladaptive schemas, coping styles, and modes. See Schema; Schema modes; Young, Jeffrey, E.; Young Schema Questionnaire.

SCHIZO Split.

SCHIZOAFFECTIVE DISORDER A hybrid disorder of *DSM* nosology that combines schizophrenic symptoms including delusions and hallucinations with a major affective psychosis of a manic or depressive nature. See Psychosis; Schizophrenia.

SCHIZOID As in the schizophrenic split of the personality. Also referred to as a split between intellectual and emotional components of the personality.

SCHIZOID PERSONALITY A personality or character disorder largely expressed by a remoteness and aloofness in interpersonal situations as well as in general demeanor. Is an Axis II personality disorder in *DSM* nomenclature. Not a psychosis. See Personality / character disorder.

SCHIZOID POSITION See Klein, Melanie.

SCHIZOPHASIA Word salad seen in the associations of some schizophrenic patients. See Word salad.

SCHIZOPHRENIA A psychosis known clinically as a thinking disorder. Includes the presence of delusions and hallucinations and disturbances in general cognitive abilities. Historically, Bleuler's four *A*s were required for this diagnosis to be made: associational disturbances (thinking and language), autism (highly idiosyncratic abnormal functioning), ambivalence (loss of adequate discriminating ability), and affect disturbance (flat affect or lability). Usual types include

Catatonic type—motoric inability in the form of catalepsy (with waxy flexibility and stupor), mutism and negativistic attitude and behavior, posturing with bizarre positions, and explosiveness (catatonic excitement).

Chronic undifferentiated schizophrenia—also referred to as mixed schizophrenia because of the appearance of symptoms typical of several of the other types of schizophrenia.

Disorganized type—disorganized speech, behavior, and affect.

Paranoid type—characterized by delusions of grandiosity or persecution and hallucinations.

Residual schizophrenia—episodic schizophrenic symptoms appear.

Past psychiatric nosology has identified the following schizophrenic types.

Hebephrenic—in which the person will exhibit childish silliness, inappropriate laughing, and like mannerisms; carries a poor (guarded) prognosis.

Simple—in which the main characteristic is a dimming of responses along with flat affect.

Variation of schizophrenic disorders include:

Acute schizophrenia—lack of insight and auditory hallucinations are classic symptoms.

Ambulatory schizophrenia—refers to a person who has been diagnosed schizophrenic but does not require hospitalization, nonetheless behaving with overpersonalized and odd ideation.

Catastrophic schizophrenia—severe schizophrenic condition immediately dissembling the personality.

Induced schizophrenia—seems to be imposed on the subject by forceful family figures.

Latent schizophrenia—symptoms exist, although there is no reality break.

Pseudoneurotic schizophrenia—See Pseudoneurotic schizophrenia.

Schizoaffective disorder—See Schizoaffective disorder.

Schizophreniform disorder—See Schizophreniform disorder.

Arieti, Cancro, Meyer, Zilboorg, and Zubin represent the legion of contributors to the investigation into the anatomy of schizophrenia.

SCHIZOPHRENIFORM DISORDER Symptoms of schizophrenia are present, but the prognosis is excellent and the person likely reconstitutes to premorbid functioning. See Schizophrenia.

SCHIZOPHRENOGENIC MOTHER The parent who engineers the flowering of schizophrenia, presumably a disturbed mother. Concept promoted by Frieda Fromm-Reichmann. The idea that the mother can convey a schizophrenic psychogenic so-called germ that then gets played out in the schizophrenically developed personality of the child.

SCHIZOTYPAL DISORDER See Personality / character disorder.

SCHOOL PHOBIA Equivalent to school refusal syndrome. See Phobia.

SCHOOL REFUSAL SYNDROME. Essentially meaning school phobia. See Phobia.

SCHORE, ALLAN (1943–). American neuroscientist and psychologist / psychoanalyst. His groundbreaking contributions have impacted the fields of psychoanalysis, affective neuroscience, neuropsychiatry, trauma theory, developmental psychology, attachment theory, pediatrics, infant mental health, psychotherapy, behavioral biology, and clinical social work. Known for his interdisciplinary perspective, his activities as a clinical scientist span from his theoretical work on the enduring impact of early trauma on brain development, to neuroimaging research on the neurobiology of attachment and studies of borderline personality disorder, to his biological studies of relational trauma in wild elephants, to his practice of psychotherapy.

SCHREBER CASE Freud's analysis of the profile of a man with paranoid delusions in which a theoretical connection was made between the paranoid delusional state and a presumed underlying homosexual wish.

SCOPOPHILIA The experience of pleasure in the act of looking and thus a component of voyeurism. See Voyeur or Voyeurism.

SCREEN Referred to in dream theory as a screen dream, where one person can substitute for another and the screen is the substitute figure that becomes central in the dream. See Screen memory.

SCREEN MEMORY In psychoanalytic usage this refers to using a specific memory as a screen or block that conceals a memory of a more significant event, one that is likely to involve another implicated person. In addition, the screen memory can be interpreted as a symbolic illustration of personal conflict.

SEARLES, HAROLD F. (1918–). American psychiatrist/psychoanalyst who is known, among many other contributions, for the examination of countertransference understanding in the treatment of borderline and psychotic subjects.

SEASONAL AFFECTIVE DISORDER Known as winter depression. Reported to be ameliorated by artifical light. May also be a function of a reduction of Vitamin D due to the absence of sufficient sunlight in winter.

SECONDARY ELABORATION See Dream theory, Freudian.

SECONDARY GAIN See Gain, secondary.

SECONDARY PROCESS Behavior mediated by the ego and reality testing, where impulses are calibrated accordingly, with consciousness prevailing so that instincts from the unconscious are unlikely to gain the ascendancy. See Frontal lobe executive control systems; Primary process; Thinking.

SECURITY OPERATIONS Conceptualized by Sullivan to indicate that the person engages in many emotional experiences, as in the expression of anger or even contempt, in the service of managing anxiety.

SELECTIVE ABSTRACTION In Beck's cognitive theory, reflects cognitive bias so that the individual increases both selective perception (sees what s/he wants to see) as well as perceptual defense (doesn't see what s/he doesn't want to see). See Automatic thoughts; Beck, Aaron T.

SELECTIVE MUTISM A social anxiety disorder. See Mutism, elective.

SELECTIVE SEROTONIN REUPTAKE INHIBITORS (SSRIS) Antidepressants for depression, personality, and anxiety disorders. See Antidepressant medications; Serotonin.

SELF In psychoanalytic usage, equivalent to ego and composed of both conscious and unconscious elements. Implicit in the work of Aron, on one- and two-person psychologies, and in the work of Ghent.

SELF, BAD referring to the phenomenon of projection onto the other of negative attributes one unconsciously assigns to the self.

SELF, FALSE See Winnicott, D. W.

SELF, TRUE Through the psychoanalytic process, the surfacing of unconscious material with the ultimate aim of creating a new synthesis—a truer reflection of the self. See Winnicott, D. W.

SELF-EFFACEMENT Karen Horney's concept of the person who seeks to be dependent and clinging, but is more deeply motivated by self-hate.

SELF-ESTEEM Other than feeling good about the self, in psychoanalytic terms, self-esteem is the ego's good relationship with the superego.

SELF-MUTILATION Inflicting injury on the self is the denotative meaning of self-mutilation. Psychodynamically, however, self-mutilation is seen as a symptomatic means of relieving tension, self-defeating though it is. Cutting and cigarette burning are often seen in such persons. Psychoanalytically understood as a function of severe superego introjection of parental attitudes and/or as an attempt to alleviate feelings of guilt. Unconscious feelings of anger toward the introjected figure is more fundamental here. Thus the alleviation of the guilt is really an alleviation of repressed feelings of anger, existing consciously as a vague feeling of "wrongness" about the self. Usually seen in the borderline diagnosis and related to the oedipal conflict. Occurring with women who, as with trichotillomania (hair pulling), find themselves implicated in the oedipal seduction drama.

SELFOBJECT A key concept of self psychology, in which one's estimate of self is established through the relationship of self to object and such interaction thereby sustains and contributes to the sense of selfhood.

SELFOBJECT FUNCTIONS Derived by Kohut to support the possibility of restitutive personality development. These are

idealization—provides sense of security;
mirroring—provides affirmation and validation;
twinship—provides a sense of belonging.

SELFOBJECT NEEDS Refers to an internalization concept essential for the development and sustaining nature of a positive sense of self. See Self psychology.

SELFOBJECT TRANSFERENCE Affirmation by the therapist can lead to an elevated sense of self. See Self psychology.

SELF PSYCHOLOGY Originally developed by Heinz Kohut with antecedent influence from Freud and Jung. Kohut included the psychology of empathy insofar as a person's sense of self is largely influenced by the responsiveness of others, especially with respect to the extent of empathic response. Therapeutic benefit is gained through the selfobject transference in which thwarted developmental needs for mirroring, idealizing, and alterego experiences can be regained. Thus tension reduction as the sine qua non of working through conflict recedes in importance, as does the entire oedipal issue—all in favor of the work related to the incremental maturation of the self—especially through selfobject relationships. A sample of theoreticians / clinicians who have contributed to the domain of self psychology include Bacal, Buirski, Goldberg, Josephs, Lichtenberg, A. Ornstein, P. Ornstein, Stern, and Wolf. See Kohut, Heinz.

SELF-REPRESENTATION In the psychology of the self, this refers to the ways in which the self is presented in the world in relation to others. Internalized self-representations occur when individuation is developed along with the appearance of autonomous ego functions.

SELIGMAN, MARTIN (1942–). American psychologist. Known for his work in positive psychology (the study of optimum functioning) and learned helplessness.

SELYE, HANS (1907–1982). European-born Canadian endocrinologist. Formulated the general adaptation syndrome. Influenced thinking in the psychology of stress. See General adaptation syndrome (GAS).

SEMICONSCIOUS Quasi conscious, meaning vaguely conscious.

SEMINAL EMISSION An ejaculation during sleep based upon a sexual dream. Also referred to as a wet dream.

SENESCENCE An aging phenomenon based upon genetic factors as one enters later years.

SENILITY An aging phenomenon that emphasizes environmental causes for decline or dementia in later years.

SENIUM Old age.

SENIUM PRAECOX Premature old age under sixty years.

SENSATIONAL TYPE See Jung, Carl Gustav.

SENSORIMOTOR INTELLIGENCE Piaget's observation of the first two years of the child's life, when symbolization begins, especially with respect to language and behavioral expression. The child also practices the use of muscles and senses, all in the service of understanding the world. See Piaget, Jean.

SENSORIUM The seat of sensation. In the psychiatric interview, if the subject is responding normally to surroundings (i.e., time, place, person, and memory), the psychiatric profile will indicate that the sensorium is clear.

SEPARATION ANXIETY Usually applied to separation fears of the child from the mother, but also relevant to adults who can experience this sort of separation tension in a variety of situations and relationships. More intense with individuals who are dependent personalities. Also a phenomenon that, when occurring at an age-appropriate time, is expected and normal.

SEPARATION-INDIVIDUATION PHASE See Mahler, Margaret.

SEQUELA The more permanent residue of a trauma or disorder. An example would be a facial tic that remains after the experience of extreme tension. The residual symptom, such as the tic, may be temporary.

SEROTONIN A neurotransmitter of nerve impulses. Plays an important function in the regulation of anger and aggression. Low levels produce an increase of anger and aggression.

SEXUAL DISORDERS In the psychiatric nomenclature, sexual disorders include

paraphilias—sexual deviations;
sexual dysfunction—examples are impotence and frigidity.

SEXUAL DYSFUNCTION In the psychiatric nomenclature, sexual dysfunctions include:

orgasm disorders—inhibited orgasm, premature ejaculation;
sexual arousal disorder—equivalent to impotence and frigidity;
sexual aversion disorder—aversion to sexual activity;
sexual pain disorder—genital pain, vaginismus.

See Vaginismus.

SEXUAL INVERSION A Freudian concept regarding homosexuality in which variation of sexual orientation can be seen.

SEXUALITY Other than commonsense interest in sex and sexual role identity, sexuality has played an important role in psychoanalytic theory. Freud considered psychic energy connected to somatic satisfaction to be the emotional chemistry of sexuality, which he termed the instinct of Eros, related for the most part to self-preservation. In addition, Freud postulated the sexually associated phases of child development in his infantile psychosexual stages of oral, anal, phallic, and oedipal.

Sex role—those attitudes and behavioral correlates that are usually more associated with one gender and less or not at all with the other.
Sex role inversion—identifying with the opposite sex.

SEXUALITY, INFANTILE A psychoanalytic concept referring to pleasure derived in childhood from erotogenic zones.

SEXUAL ORIENTATION Usually either heterosexual or homosexual.

SEXUAL RESPONSE CYCLE Generally the cycle includes initial *fantasy* (or attraction), leading to *excitement,* in turn leading to *orgasm,* then to *resolution* (relaxation).

SHADOW Jung's definition of the unconscious in which resides the sum of all of a person's negative qualities that are deemed necessary to conceal.

SHAMAN A person identified as a healer who claims either supernatural or extranatural powers.

SHAME Shame is understood from a number of vantage points:

Personality-trait perspective—conceptualized as composed of the emotions of sorrow, disgust, and fear. This means that the person feels a loss of esteem (sorrow about), an inclination to flee (fear), and a sense of humiliation (disgust).

Psychoanalytic perspective—Shame is thought to be correlated with the anal / phallic psychosexual stage of conflict insofar as there may be difficulties (that are usually exaggerated) during toilet training, creating implications for the development of a lower threshold of experiencing shame as well as anxiety concerning assertion. Derivative issues such as the ambition drive (a derivative of the phallic phase) is considered the person's antidote or defense against shame, insofar as the expectation of ambition / success sustains self-esteem.

Self-psychology perspective—Shame is considered the fount or source of influence on the entire spectrum of emotions. In this sense, shame is seen as the basis of humiliation and self-loathing and is therefore, according to this view, profoundly related to the sense of self. Contributors to the understanding of the psychology and vicissitudes of shame include H. B. Lewis and A. P. Morrison.

SHAM RAGE See Rage, sham.

SHAPING In behavior therapy, reinforcing successive approximations as a means of gradually achieving desired behavior.

SHARED PARANOID DISORDER A psychosis in which two people in a folie à deux show the same paranoid symptoms. Referred to in *DSM* nomenclature as shared psychotic disorder.

SHELDON, WILLIAM HERBERT (1899–1977). American psychologist best known for his body typology (somatotype) and its relation to personality (temperament).

Somatotype	*Temperament*
Ectomorph—thin and edgy.	Cerebrotonia—inhibited.
Endomorph—rotund and jovial.	Viscerotonia—needs for affection.
Mesomorph—athletic and stable.	Somatotonia—assertive need.

Included in the typology system is a scale so that various extents related to each type can be assessed.

SHELL SHOCK Combat neurosis to trauma of war. Subsumed under the diagnosis of posttraumatic stress syndrome arising from a battle situation.

SHOCK TREATMENT Shocking the central nervous system as in the use of electroconvulsive therapy (ECT). See Electroconvulsive therapy (ECT).

SHORT-TERM MEMORY Usually an organic impairment leading to a loss of recent past memory—even that of an elapsed minute.

SIBLING RIVALRY The competition among brothers and sisters.

SIDE EFFECT Usually referring to drug reactions that are not the aim of the medication, but rather a deleterious extraneous effect.

SIGNAL ANXIETY A Freudian concept indicating the anticipatory anxiety that forewarns of impending danger. Originally the anticipated danger was thought to be from threatening impulses (forbidden wishes) within, but was later broadened to a more general sense of danger about to be triggered. By means of signal anxiety, mechanisms to prevent and avoid the arousal of further anxiety and feelings that would be considered threatening or dangerous are avoided by the mobilization of various defensive maneuvers. These include defense mechanisms and character traits designed to keep the feelings sensed as dangerous at bay. Such a defensive reaction prevents the emergence of feelings that are anticipated as painful, humiliating, or overwhelming that would create in a drop in self-esteem. As a result, a range of emotions are not experienced nor realistically integrated into the person's broader adaption, but the person is spared the full-blown and more general experience of discomfort by responding to the alarm function that signal anxiety represents. Analogous to Pavlov's conditioned response. See Anxiety.

SILVER CORD SYNDROME A family constellation with an especially passive father and exceedingly controlling mother thought to be etiologically a contributing cause of schizophrenia or psychosexual identity shift or such self-same pathology in a latent, prodromal, or virtual state.

SIMPLE SCHIZOPHRENIA See Schizophrenia.

SKINNER, B. F. (Burrhus Frederic; 1904–1990). Prominent American psychologist who originated operant conditioning and was instrumental in the development of the field of applied behavioral analysis, the application of his ideas to educational methods, child rearing, and psychotherapy, among others. His most famous books include *Behavior of Organisms* and *Walden Two.* See Reinforcement.

SLABY, ANDREW (1942–). American psychiatrist and epidemiologist. Author and editor. Specialist in stress management and depression. Professor of psychiatry, New York University Medical Center, and former president, American Association of Suicidology. Member, editorial board, *Dictionary of Psychopathology.*

SLAVSON, S. R. (1890–1981). European-born American psychologist. Prominent influential pioneer in the modality of group therapy. See Group therapy.

SLEEP Consisting of nondream sleep (NREM), and dream sleep (REM: rapid eye movement). A normal cycle of sleep begins with stage 1, which is light sleep, then progresses to a deeper sleep, stage 2, moving to a still deeper sleep, stage 3, and reaching D sleep, or deepest sleep, stage 4. After stage 4, sleep lightens and REM dreaming begins. This completes the first cycle, followed again by the beginning of the next cycle. Each cycle lasts about ninety minutes. See Sleep disorders.

SLEEP APNEA Respiratory disturbance (obstruction) that interrupts sleep and causes daytime drowsiness because of this distress of nighttime sleep. Such interruptions are essentially a condition in which, for short durations, breathing ceases. See SAHS-UAO.

SLEEP DISORDERS Consisting of four general categories:

DIMS or disorders of initiating and maintaining sleep—also referred to as the *dyssomnias*. These are the insomnias and include variations of excessive daytime sleepiness.

The sleep-wake schedule disorders—these include those variations of sleepiness during times when others are awake and the opposite tendency of feeling awake when one should be asleep. Also known as circadian rhythm sleep disorder, considered a dyssomnia.

Parasomnias—including night terrors, sleepwalking, nightmares, and sleep paralysis. See Parasomnia.

Disorder of excessive somnolence (DOES)—excessive lag time between sleep and wakefulness. Confusion along with aggression may occur during the wakefulness phase. Seen in males and referred to as sleep drunkenness.

Other sleep disorder phenomena:

Hypersomnia—excessive sleep.

Hypersomnolence disorder—excessive sleep along with the absence of refreshing sleep, as in naps.

Narcolepsy—excessive daytime sleepiness. See Narcolepsy.

Sleep drunkenness—disorder of excessive somnolence.

Sleep terror disorder—pavor nocturnes or night terror. Seen in children who awaken screaming in terror. Occurring generally during stage 3 or 4 of the sleep cycle, meaning in non-REM (NREM) sleep (or nondream sleep).

SLEEP DRUNKENNESS See Sleep Disorders.

SLEEP INVERSION Usually defined as sleeping by day, feeling awake at night.

SLEEP LATENCY The time elapsing between trying to sleep and actual sleep. See Sleep disorders.

SLEEP TERROR DISORDER See Sleep Disorders.

SLIP OF THE TONGUE A Freudian observation that has been made popular, alluding to an unconscious verbalization unintended by the subject but implying some true sentiment that was ostensibly covert and defended against. See Parapraxis.

SOCIALIZATION Becoming integrated in society in a normal manner; obeying laws of civility. In a psychoanalytic sense, meaning the ability to govern one's impulses in conformity to the conditions of external reality demands.

SOCIAL PHOBIA Extreme reluctance to enter social situations. See Phobia.

SOCIAL RELEASER Any stimulus that releases instinctive behavior.

SOCIAL STRESSOR Life events that are important benchmarks in a person's life or that comprise crisis situations.

SOCIOBIOLOGY The presumed biological/genetic underpinning to personality traits, motivation, and behavior, also containing epigenetic imperatives. See Epigenesis.

SOCIOPATH Antisocial personality. See Psychopathic personality.

SODOMY Anal intercourse.

SOFT SIGNS Referring to diagnostic signs that are only suggestive of the particular diagnosis but not of the hard-core sign of the diagnosis, or what is known as a pathognomonic sign.

SOILING See Encopresis.

SOLIPSISM Ego above all. Philosophically, it is the person's sense that all knowledge is known through the self. Psychoanalytically, in maladaptive form, is considered to be narcissistic preoccupation.

SOLMS, MARK (1961–). South African–born neuropsychologist and psychoanalyst credited as the founder of the field of neuropsychoanalysis. Investigated the brain mechanisms of emotion, motivation, and the psychological mechanisms of confabulation and anosognosia syndromes. Interested in defining consciousness from a brain/biology vantage point and best known for his discovery of the forebrain mechanisms of dreaming.

SOMA Referring to the body, in contrast to the mind or psyche.

SOMATIZATION Essentially converting tension and neurotic conflict into bodily symptoms known as psychosomatic or psychophysiological symptoms.

SOMATOFORM DISORDERS Those bodily disorders for which there is no medical basis.

Body dysmorphic disorder—the imagining of a defect of the body and pursuing treatment avenues when all medical evidence is negative. See Dysmorphophobia.

Conversion (hysteria) disorder—appearance of an actual physical defect that has its basis in a neurotic psychological conversion to a physical symptom. See Conversion and conversion hysteria.

Hypochondriasis—misinterpreting a bodily sensation and believing in the presence of a serious disease. See Hypochondriasis.

Somatization disorder—history of somatic complaints requiring frequent medical examinations without any tangible evidence of physical impairment.

Somatoform pain disorder—complaints of severe pain leading to extreme medical applications and what is known as "doctor shopping."

SOMNAMBULISM See sleepwalking.

SOMNOLENCE Continued drowsiness.

SOPORIFIC Sleep-inducing agent.

SOTERIA Any collectible item or object the person has and about which the person feels secure, insofar as the proximity of the object provides reassurance—in the sense of a deliverance. Analogous to any transitional object, such as a child's favorite blanket, that offers a sense of security and safety. See Winnicott, D. W.

SOUL Usually considered to be one's true self. Jung's concept of anima.

SPITZ, RENE A. (1887–1974). European-born American psychoanalyst who studied child development, concentrating on the first year of life. He identified "critical periods" that suggested a fixed program of development as well as noting the development of ego maturation. His work corresponds to that of Mahler and Hartmann with respect to the underpinning of ego psychology and the merging of the biological and psychological. Studied depression in its relation to the experience of psychological abandonment. Results from the impoverishment of affectional needs during the first year of life were then termed anaclitic depression. Also studied stranger anxiety. See Anaclitic depression.

SPLIT PERSONALITY See dissociative identity disorder.

SPLITTING A defense mechanism of the psyche that manages inner tension by compartmentalization. In this sense, the person can identify objects as good or bad or can idealize or demonize (devalue) others. Thus, instead of the ability to see positive as well as negative traits in a person (enabling a synthesis), the object can be "split" into good and bad, thus avoiding the tension of ambivalence. Popularized in the object relations literature by Melanie Klein. See Klein, Melanie.

SPOTNITZ, HYMAN (1908–2008). American psychiatrist who differed from Freud with respect to the probability of treating schizophrenic and narcissistic disorders psychoanalytically. Freud eschewed such practice with these diagnostic types, while Spotnitz's position was that such disorders could be, in fact, reversed. Spotnitz is the founder of what he termed modern psychoanalysis.

SPOUSAL ABUSE Typical of a husband abusing a wife—usually by physically harming her. Also referred to as wife beating or wife battering. Thought to be a function of the husband's need for esteem and control based upon a deeper sense of inadequacy. He will also be particularly subject to jealous rage. Seeking compensatory adoration but perceiving the opposite can set off eruptive, aggressive, and assaultive behavior in such ego-weak individuals. See Shame.

SQUIGGLE GAME See Winnicott, D. W.

STAGE FRIGHT A performer's intense fear of appearing before a live audience. Attributed psychoanalytically to castration fears or to the variation of this fear—that the audience will see a person of the opposite sex or, rather, be able to ascertain certain guilts.

STAMMERING Spasmodic speech disorder.

STANFORD-BINET INTELLIGENCE SCALE Intelligence test predating the Wechsler Scales that assesses intelligence and cognitive abilities. Includes verbal, nonverbal, and full-scale scores and is used with children and adults from early childhood through advanced years (ages two through eighty-nine). Developed by Alfred Binet, a French psychologist (1857–1911) who, later, with Theodore Simon, published the Binet-Simon test, eventually to be revised by Lewis Terman, a Stanford psychologist, and published in revised version as the Stanford-Binet Intelligence Test.

STEALING SPLURGE Referring to children who steal, presumably as a compensatory need for power and prestige and, from a psychoanalytic point of view, as a way of becoming an oedipal winner—by stealing the prize (opposite-sex parent).

STEKEL, WILHELM (1868–1940). European physician and psychologist who has influenced the field of active psychotherapy as a possible way to shorten the therapeutic process.

STEREOTYPED MOVEMENT DISORDERS A childhood disorder (mostly seen in boys) characterized by involuntary motility or tics:

chronic motor tic disorder—involving three or fewer muscle groups;
Tourette's disorder—wide variety of bodily and vocal tics;
transient tic disorder—usually a facial tic;
miscellaneous—head banging and rocking.

See Tic.

STEREOTYPY Clinically referring to repetitive behavior resembling a tic.

STERILITY Barrenness or infertility.

STIGMATA Localized marks (Christian history). Psychoanalytically considered to be a conversion somatization symptom with a libidinous underpinning and can be seen as an attempt to spiritualize hysteria.

STIMULUS CONTROL Behavior therapy technique involving arranging the environment in such a way that a given response is either more or less likely to occur (e.g., keeping binge foods out of the house; staying away from bars).

STIMULUS TENSION Freud's phrase for tension that is generated by a stimulus.

STIMULUS WORD A particular word utilized in tests of association.

STOCK-STILL BEHAVIOR A developmental marker at about age seventeen and a half months. In the absence of any hesitation, toddlers will stop motionless at the entranceway to previously traversed nursery room. Presumably signals an awareness of self/object differentiation and suggests an increase in body awareness. Theoretically connected to the psychoanalytic concept of anal phase behavior. A sample of theoreticians interested in the study of this behavior includes Fonagy, Sherkow, and Weinstein.

STOLOROW, ROBERT (1942–). American psychologist/psychoanalyst. Founding member, Institute of Contemporary Psychoanalsysis and Institute for the Psychoanalytic Study of Subjectivity. Member, editorial board, *Dictionary of Psychopathology.* Originator, with George Atwood and later Bernard Brandchaft and Donna Orange, of the intersubjective perspective in psychoanalysis, based upon a general theory of subjectivity. The subjective experience at the intersection of therapist and patient constitutes a contextualization that, with respect to developmental and psychoanalytic theory, is the basis for a new synthesis in the specific psychotherapeutic event as well as process. The reciprocal interaction between patient and therapist becomes the closest reality in this endeavor, that is, that personal experience gains its configuration in the context of interrelatedness. See Intersubjectivity theory.

STRANGER ANXIETY Normal part of development whereby the child experiences distress when confronted with unfamiliar people. Signs include hiding behind a parent, crying, withdrawing by turning the head away, and staring. Can occur as early as six months, but usually appears between eight or nine months and begins to disappear after about one year of age. After a year and a half, a sustained reaction of stranger anxiety signals a more serious problem and implies a need for diagnostic assessment regarding a possible developmental disorder.

STREAM OF CONSCIOUSNESS The patient's free associational narrative sequence.

STRESS Perhaps the most ubiquitous "normal" psychopathology. A reaction of the individual to disturbing stimuli as applied to all people. Psychologically, however, Kellerman proposes that the culprit for that which causes stress concerns either conscious, subconscious, or repressed anger. Whether a low-intensity annoyance such as boredom, which may cause stress, or a high-intensity dissatisfaction, which will also cause stress, these may be a disguised lexicon for the presence of anger—albeit repressed anger. When a person's wish is thwarted—either the escape from boredom is blocked or a major wish is blocked—a loss of power becomes a normal reaction. This, in turn, will generate anger because where there is disempowerment, or a sense of the absence of some ability to express one's prerogative (i.e., a measure of helplessness), becoming angry may be the only immediate path to reempowerment. Therefore, assuming the veracity of this hypothesis regarding stress and its relation to anger, any stress may be associated to its more specific problem—the presence of anger (conscious or not). Hans Selye's general adaptation syndrome, in which the subject experiences an alarm reaction, then a resistance to the alarm that ushers in an adaptation to it (albeit with much energy expenditure), then general exhaustion, has been the historical approach in the understanding of stress. The salient tone in each of the phases of the general adaptation syndrome—alarm, resistance, and exhaustion—is that of the person's anger and its vicissitudes. Usually, these are disguised in the syntactical form identified as stress. The alarm stage, which is a shock to the system plus a compensatory attempt to regain one's footing, may actually be the person feeling suddenly disempowered, surprised by it, thus instantly angry. Second, the resistance stage, when the person tries to restabilize, can be considered an attempt to regain some reempowerment by feeling angry. Third, the exhaustion stage, where symptoms can include sleeplessness, loss of appetite, irritability, and fatigue, is already a pathognomic indication anger has been repressed and the stress already a transformed symptom and psychically gratified wish that, because it is a symptom, symbolically represents full reempowerment, and therefore psychologically this symptom represents an entire psychic restabilization—ergo Freud's promise that in the psyche no wish will be denied. See general adaptation syndrome (GAS); Symptom.

STRESS MANAGEMENT In cognitive behavior therapy, REBT, and behavior therapy, use of relaxation, breathing, and cognitive coping methods to reduce anxiety, tension, and other distressful feelings and improve functioning in the face of overload or stress-potentiating situations.

STRUCTURAL INTEGRATION See Rolfing.

STRUCTURAL PROFILE This profile is the subject's self-rating of the BASIC ID scales. See Basic ID.

STRUCTURAL THEORY One of several theories developed by Sigmund Freud. The structural theory posits the psychic structure of ego / id / superego. The ego mediates between the drives of the id and the policing agency of the superego. See Freud, Sigmund.

STRUCTURED CLINICAL INTERVIEW FOR *DSM-IV* Instrument for use to assess diagnoses of Axis I and Axis II disorders, including depressive as well as other diagnoses.

STRUCTURED FAMILY THERAPY (SFT) See Minuchin, Salvador.

STUPOR, EMOTIONAL Symptoms of emotional stupor include mutism and anxiety. Considered to be an "emotional braking" in which the brain creates the ability to halt an ostensible stampede of emotion that has begun to overwhelm the subject. This stampede of emotion is possibly the onslaught of an inexorable rage reaction. See Psychopathology; Symptom.

STUTTERING Sputtering speech disorder including halting speech.

SUBCONSCIOUSNESS Quasi consciousness.

SUBLIMATION Psychoanalytic concept of an ego process in which impulse and the libidinous life are harnessed and converted into productive work energy, instinct into noninstinct.

SUBSTITUTE FORMATION Equivalent to the notion of derivatives, a concept central to psychoanalytic inquiry. Neurotic symptoms are derivatives of source impulses and repressed material.

SUBSYMBOLIC PROCESS In intersubjectivity theory, the subsymbolic process is a nonmanipulative integration model linking emotional and verbal processing. Incorporates idea of implicit relational knowing.

SUCCESS, FAILURE THROUGH A superego imperative that prevails when the person is on the verge of success, so that the moment of impending success is renounced.

SUCCESSIVE APPROXIMATIONS The incremental steps in therapy toward the analysis of conflicts, where it is expected that the patient will make the necessary synapses connecting present to past in order to achieve resolution of conflict.

SUCCUBUS In fantasy, a female supernatural being who has sex with men while they sleep. See Incubus.

SUGGESTIBILITY Characteristic trait of hysterical personalities in which the subject is susceptible to the influence of others.

SUICIDE, PSYCHIC Killing oneself, in the absence of a physical act, through the wish to die.

SULLIVAN, HARRY STACK (1892–1949). American psychiatrist / psychoanalyst. Promoted the theory of interpersonal relationships in the study of psychopatholgy and treatment, in contrast to the conception of a biological underpinning to psychoanalysis. Some Sullivanian conceptions of consciousness and thinking include:

Dynamisms—particular thinking and behavior that characterizes the individual.

Personifications—images of oneself and others that become generalized.

Modes of experience / levels of thinking—these are types of relationships drawn between events:

- *Prototaxic mode*—in infancy, random feelings and thoughts that have no obvious connection.
- *Parataxic mode*—feelings and experiences connected correlationally.

Syntaxic mode—understanding of meaning through words.

Sullivan's defense system included

dissociation—equivalent to repression;
parataxic distortion—repetition of childhood patterns;
sublimation—undesirable behavior transformed into that which is socially acceptable.

SUNDOWNER Referring to elderly individuals who seem well functioning during the day but become less clear in the evening.

SUPEREGO Conscience and/or the agency of self-criticism. In psychoanalysis, one of three components of structural theory. The superego is essentially unconscious and stands in judgment of the ego while trying to exert influence on the id.

SUPEREGO INTERPRETATION An understanding reached by the patient regarding internal demands that are usually adhered to and contribute to the patient's masochistic tendency of self-imposed stresses.

SUPEREGO RESISTANCE See Resistance, superego.

SUPERVALENT THOUGHT See Thought disorder.

SUPPRESSION Different from repression in that suppression contains a conscious component.

SURFACE COGNITIONS Refers to descriptions, inferences, and attributes.

SURFACE EGO Freud's notion that the ego, because of its role in confronting the stimuli of the external world, exists on the surface of the psyche.

SURRENDER, WILL TO The point at which the patient's aim is congruent with the therapist's aim—to resolve the neurosis—to relinquish it. A triumph over resistance, provided that the congruence is not based on simple positive transference or the gratification experienced by the patient as a result of feeling understood, because feeling understood can also be a validation of one's defenses.

SURROGATE PARENT A person who fits the role of an ideal figure that can substitute for the parent.

SUTTIE, IAN (1889–1935). Scottish psychiatrist who challenged Freudian orthodoxy. He was arguably the first object relations theorist who rejected instinct theory and was also the first theorist to indicate a link of the self with the object that transcended drive theory. He identified selfobject functioning and, rather than relating anger to the aggressive drive, felt that anger was a demand for help. He extolled human companionship as the salient issue of human affairs. A sample of some of his key observations and postulates that relate to love and hate include

Paradigm for love—the infant is born into a nonsexual relationship with mother, and this is the basic paradigm for love.

Separation psychology—as a developmental phenomenon, a normal separation process from mother is essential, and faulty separation can lead to feelings of hate, cynicism, and pessimism.

Developmental challenge—to develop a healthy personality, it is necessary to accept and win the challenge for independence.

SYDENHAM, THOMAS (1624–1689). British physician credited with creating the classification system for diagnosis on the basis of syndromal formulations that still influence the *DSM* classification model.

SYMBIOSIS Reciprocal interdependence.

SYMBIOTIC INFANTILE PSYCHOSIS See Psychosis, symbiotic infantile.

SYMBIOTIC PHASE See Mahler, Margaret.

SYMBOL Something representing something else. In psychoanalytic dream theory, symbolization is one of the four dream mechanisms that act to translate the latent primary process material into the manifest dream so that the dream has some semblance of a story line. In addition, psychoanalytically, a symbol is also a condensation, substitution, and abstraction that references an unconscious idea or even conflict. There are several variants.

anagogic symbol—implying striving toward an ego ideal;
cryptogenic symbol—pictorial;

functional symbol—representing emotional insufficiency; *metaphoric symbol*—pictorial metaphor.

SYMBOL, PHALLIC An object that represents a penis. As a personification, a phallic man denotes that the person is assertive. Stereotypically, when the phrase is applied to a woman, it usually implies an aggressive and dominant person.

SYMBOLIC REGISTER See Lacan, Jacques-Marie-Emil.

SYMPATHETIC NERVOUS SYSTEM See Autonomic nervous system.

SYMPATHIZE To have compassion for another. See Empathy.

SYMPTOM The most representative symbol of psychopathology. In psychoanalytic understanding, a substitute for the wish. Freud saw the symptom as a compromise because of the ego's challenge of impulse and subsequent signal anxiety. His postulate that in the psyche no wish will be denied is accomplished by the appearance of the symptom. In a separate formulation, Kellerman postulates that a psychological symptom contains four terms to its formation:

1. the thwarting of a wish;
2. experiencing anger toward the "who," who thwarted the wish;
3. repression of the anger, along with the original wish; and,
4. appearance of the symptom as the perverse form of the wish.

Several axioms along with their corollaries are proposed to account for the process of symptom formation and underscore the salient issues of the symptom formation phenomenon:

Where there is a symptom, not only will there be repressed anger (along with the wish), there must be repressed anger (along with the wish);

Where there is repressed anger (along with the wish), not only will there be a symptom, there must be a symptom;

Where there is no symptom, not only will there be no repressed anger (and no repressed wish), there cannot be repressed anger (nor can there be a repressed wish);

Where there is no repressed anger (and no repressed wish), not only will there not be a symptom, there cannot be a symptom.

Therefore, the vicissitudes of anger (in relation to the who, the wish, and repression itself) become the key to understanding symptoms. That is, when the wish is thwarted, the person feels helpless or disempowered. Helplessness or disempowerment breeds anger or rage every time, in every person. Anger then frequently becomes the only way to be reempowered. The problem is that the anger is frequently repressed because the object of the anger, most often and for any number of reasons, cannot be confronted. Therefore, the subject's anger is repressed and, of course, then directed toward the self. The reason for this directing of anger toward the self concerns a basic law of emotion that reveals the phenomenon of emotion as becoming complete, or becoming realized as an emotion, only when it takes (connects to) an object (a person). In the absence of the possibility of attaching to the intended "who," the emotion (in this case, anger) then attaches to the self. When it attaches to the self, the anger will then behave accordingly, attacking the self. This attack nature of anger is the ignition that morphs the wish into the symptom (hence a gratified wish), albeit in symbolic form, as a neurotic or perverse product of the psyche. Thus Freud's formulation that we love our symptoms becomes clear, that is, that the symptom is the realized wish, albeit in translated or symbolic or perverse or neurotic form. In addition, Kellerman proposes that if the original wish is cast in a positive way (to want something) then the symptom will yield pleasure (relief of pain); cast in a negative way (to avoid something) the symptom will be painful. He also proposes that, with respect to the three therapeutic vectors of the treatment (resistance, feeling understood, and the pathology itself), it is only the application of the infrastructural understanding of the symptom that has any hope of addressing and actually defeating the pathology. Thus, the patient's sense of feeling understood by the therapist (in the context of good rapport) can cement the therapeutic relationship, but will never have real therapeutic impact on the pathology except with respect to the phenomenon of flight into health. Aggression as a critical factor in symptom formation has been addressed by a number of theoreticians, including Gaylin, Raphling, and Parens, and symptoms as appearing in the therapeutic session itself has been considered by Luborsky. See Therapeutic vectors.

SYNCHRONICITY A Jungian notion suggesting that there are coincidences that are more than mere coincidence. These are believed to be significant synapses between a psychological internal world and some external, seemingly unrelated world.

SYNCRETIC THINKING See Thinking.

SYNCRETISTIC THINKING Equivalent to paralogical thinking or correlational thinking in which cause and effect is substituted for by the correlating two disparate events. It is considered to be pathologically concrete, in contrast to the understanding of the abstraction of cause and effect. The adage is correlation is not necessarily causation. See Paleologic thinking.

SYNDROME An amalgam of symptoms that together suggest a particular pathology or a particular diagnostic category.

SYNDROME, ANGRY MAN The male counterpart to the angry woman syndrome concerns similar symptoms to that of the woman. All of these characteristics revolve around masculine pride and the need to be adored. In addition, in the male the syndrome contains narcissistic elements along with poor frustration tolerance leading to possible abusive behavior. The suicidal implications that are seen in women with this particular syndrome are absent in men—instead replaced by violent behavior. In addition, rather than the compulsive orderliness seen in women with this syndrome, in men, the assumption is made that the wife will take care of all inconvenient details, thus reflecting an infantile omniscient wish on the part of the man with a corresponding underlying dependency need along with an insistent impatience that, if not satisfied, can lead to abuse.

SYNDROME, ANGRY WOMAN Seemingly of borderline diagnosis indicating symptoms of excessive criticality, thin stimulus barrier, compulsive orderliness, intermittent explosive reactions, substance abuse, severe marital maladjustment, and even suicidal implications. Originally applied as housewife syndrome.

SYNESTHESIA Associated sensations from two different sense modalities in which one causes the other, hearing a particular sound and simultaneously seeing a color.

SYSTEMATIC DESENSITIZATION A step-by-step procedure used in behavior therapy for replacing anxiety with relaxation while gradually increasing exposure to a hierarchy of anxiety-producing situations or objects. See Wolpe, Joseph.

SYSTEMS THEORY Generally referring to the understanding of group behavior from the vantage point of measuring networks of interactions as in family dynamics, therapy groups, or larger social groups. A sample of contributors from a wide variety of scientific disciplines who have presented the value of a systems theory approach include Banathy, Bertalanffy, H. E. Durkin, J. E. Durkin, and Prigogine.

SZASZ, THOMAS (1920–). Hungarian-born American psychiatrist / psychoanalyst. Staunch defender of patient's rights. Challenged definitions of mental illness and the existence of mental illness itself. Libertarian whose criticism of the authoritarianism of the institutionalized psychiatric establishment is legion. Strictly opposed to coercion, which he felt was the underpinning to the power of the psychiatric establishment. Prolific writer. Author of the classic volume, *The Myth of Mental Illness*.

SZONDI, LEOPOLD (1893–1986). European psychiatrist who believed that genes determine mate selection. Developer of the Szondi Test.

SZONDI TEST A projective test in which subjects are given photographs of faces and asked to choose those liked least and those liked most. Personality dimensions assessed include homosexual / sadistic, epileptic / hysterical, catatonic / paranoid, and depressive / manic.

T

T-GROUP *T* for task. The T-group is a task-oriented learning group with a definite aim and usually a time-limited framework. It is not an ongoing therapy group.

TABULA RASA Blank or clean slate. Clinically, an example is the newborn child or the mind of the newborn.

TACIT KNOWLEDGE Implicit or unconscious knowledge acquired in the absence of specific study (knowledge not formally taught, i.e., social rules). Rather, the knowledge is present through the acquisition of culture and social regulation and stored therefore without awareness. Tacit knowledge helps individuals to succeed in certain environments. See Cognitive unconscious.

TANGENTIAL SPEECH Seen in schizophrenic language in which the subject consistently strays from the main point but refers to it in a peripheral way.

TARDIVE DYSKINESIA Involuntary ticlike behavior around the oral cavity, mouth, lips, face, or even vocal chords as a result of the ingestion of large amounts of psychotropic medications, including high doses and overdoses, over long periods of time. Considered difficult or even impossible to cure. It is a neurological disorder that can also cause rapid movements of the extremities, eye blinking, tongue protrusion, or any number of other such behaviors.

TAT (THEMATIC APPERCEPTION TEST) One of the widely used standard tests of the projective battery, designed by Murray and Morgan. The subject is presented a series of pictures that depict ambiguous situations. Instructions are to imagine what describes the current scene, what was the past of the scene (what led up to it), and what the future holds. Interpretation is made with respect to interpersonal dynamics as well as to the person's sense of potential to engage the world with effort. For example, the absence of effort to attain goals in the stories implies magical thinking and, therefore, immaturity. Further, interpretation of the stories permits an analysis of the person's psychological profile, such as the ability to conduct relationships, to control aggression, and the nature of the subject's self-esteem and identity, generally revealing elements of diagnostic importance such as the presence of depression, paranoia, or any number of other personality dispositions. See Projective test battery.

TEA AND TOAST SYNDROME Applied to elderly individuals who are somewhat depressed and who, therefore, both out of depression as well as from a diminished sense of motivation, begin to subsist on very little.

TELEOLOGICAL REGRESSION Referring to Adler's theoretical underpinning in his individual psychology, in which the patient's personal goals become essential in the pursuit of the success of the treatment. *Teleological* refers to the purpose of a goal.

TELEPATHY A term used to claim a reading of minds or the transmission of messages through directed thinking or what is called channeling.

TEMPER TANTRUM The eruptive behavior (usually of a child) emanating out of frustration. Considered clinically to be regressive behavior that contraindicates the ability to postpone gratification. Instead, immediate needs for gratification, considered to be immature, dominate the moment.

TEMPERAMENT A mood disposition. Inclined toward a certain emotional tone as a characteristic of the personality.

TENSION Clinically, a more general way to refer to anxiety.

TERROR Intense fear. A lower-intensity level of fear would be "apprehension." Thus, on an intensity scaling dimension, apprehension, fear, and terror would represent a low, middle, and high level of the entire fear emotion spectrum.

TERROR, NIGHT See Night terror.

THANATOS In Freudian theory, thanatos is the death instinct.

THERAPEUTIC COMMUNITY Usually referring to nonhospital residential treatment centers.

THERAPEUTIC REGRESSION A phenomenon seen in psychoanalytic psychotherapy in which the patient, through transferential and free associational experiences, recedes or regresses to an earlier level of functioning.

Such regression is presumably in the service of the ego and ultimately leads to a better synthesis of the person's personality organization. See Regression in the service of the ego.

THERAPEUTIC VECTORS According to Kellerman, in the treatment process there are three powerful vectors defined as the resistance, the feeling of being understood, and the pathology itself.

- *resistance*—can be the weakest of the three, even though the patient can feel understood by the analyst. This vector is important because the resistance (subject to therapeutic work) is the major line of support for repression. Therefore, with resistance receding, access to repressed material (both with respect to free association as well as to interpretation) becomes more likely.
- *Feeling understood*—the defeat of a certain amount of resistance by the experience of feeling understood is never enough to have any really profound impact on the pathology itself. Yet feeling understood can relax resistance. Feeling understood is the effect on the patient of the therapist's empathy. The empathy is what is delivered; correspondingly, the patient's gratitude is what is meant by feeling understood. Although feeling understood will lower resistance to the work, the presenting psychopathology will nevertheless be sustained. On the negative side, feeling understood can also reinforce existing defenses and character structure so that no matter "how you are" can feel as though "it's OK."
- *Pathology*—is only lightly touched by the subject feeling understood as well as by the relaxation of resistance. In conventional psychodynamic psychotherapy, cure of psychopathology requires "on target" transferential working through (patient to therapist) as well as an understanding of the infrastructure of psychopathology generally and psychological symptoms specifically. See Symptoms.

THERAPIST NEUTRALITY Historically, a psychoanalytic precept. Essentially refers to the therapist's awareness that personal wishes for the patient on the part of the therapist can unconsciously bias the treatment, and short-circuit any deepening of the transferential circumstance. Such short-circuiting would be akin to partialing out of the therapy equation any negative expressions toward the therapist. In addition, it is thought that neutrality on the part of the therapist facilitates projections by the patient that can be useful in the treatment.

THIN STIMULUS BARRIER Referring to those individuals who demonstrate a poor ability to tolerate frustration. Based upon an underdevelopment of a more solid ego that would ordinarily contain necessary shock abaters in the interaction with external stimuli. Vividly seen in the borderline personality, insofar as individuals with this particular diagnosis of "borderline" find it difficult to manage their frustration and therefore exhibit frequent, though intermittent, eruptive behaviors. Also reflective of those individuals who are specifically diagnosed with intermittent eruptive or explosive disorder (IED).Also seen in individuals who have a "hot stove reaction" to some previous experience and will therefore no longer touch the "stove": for example, people who never marry because of some previous untoward family experiences or who have married but find managing the frustration and dissatisfaction with a spouse's personality too difficult, the difficulty experienced as trauma, so that to remarry becomes impossible. See Intermittent explosive disorder (IED).

THING, THE A Lacanian concept. It is lost and governed by the introduction of language and is therefore the last object to be relocated—the lost mother. It is the thing that causes the subject to speak.

THING PRESENTATION A Lacanian concept. The thing presentation is the cathexis of an idea, wish, or memory. It has word presentations corresponding to it, which, when made congruent with the "thing presentation," makes it possible for the idea, wish, or memory to be conscious.

THINKING The part of cognitive functioning that occupies the greatest amount of commonality within the cognitive parameters, that is, implicit in all forms of cognitive functions.

Abstract thinking—in development, abstract thinking reflects the most advanced form of thinking. It is the ability to generalize and to analogize.

Archaic thinking—typical of regressive schizophrenia as in "schizophrenic stupor."

Concrete thinking—the child concretizes objects but does not necessarily generalize them.

Concretistic thinking—See Syncretistic thinking.

Janusian thinking—named after Janus, the Roman god who could look in opposite directions simultaneously. Considered vital for creative thinking insofar as the creative moment is one in which opposite ideas within the parameters of any conceptual framework are accessible.

Magical thinking—See Magical thinking.

Physiognomic / syncretic thinking—the child's earliest attempt to interact with an object, even though the child may indiscriminately name it. Noted by Piaget and considered the most primitive form of thinking.

Preconscious thinking—pictorial thinking preceding logical construction. Formulated by Fenichel.

Syncretistic thinking—See Syncretistic thinking.

In addition, other more familiar references to types of thinking include:

Autistic thinking—characterized by a disregard for space and time, along with a focus on primitive wish fulfillment.

Obsessional thinking—characterized by a pervasive ambivalence.

Schizophrenic thinking—characterized by eruptions of primary process material that interfere with secondary process. In other words, cause and effect logic is severely compromised and contaminated.

In the domain of neuropsychoanalysis, aspects of thinking have been considered in a number of ways:

Unconscious and emotional thinking—according to Solms and Turnbull, such thinking is based in the limbic system.

Secondary process reality-oriented thinking—related to functions of the frontal lobe executive control systems; conscious decisions, according to Westen and others, are generated by the limbic system via emotions that are unconscious.

Primary process thinking—dreams and confabulations are manifestations of the loss of frontal executive control of mesocortical and mesolimbic "seeking" systems.

In the domain of neuropsychoanalysis, and according to Schore, in line with Freud's speculation that the primary process system emerges in human infancy before the secondary process system, the early-maturing emotional right brain is the seat of primary process, while the late developing verbal left brain organizes secondary process cognition. Schore further argues that the primary process system includes affects, imagery, metaphors, and nonverbal communication that depict an individual's relation with the social environment. This primary process communication is essential to both the attachment and psychotherapy contexts and includes body movements, posture, gesture, facial expression, voice inflection, and the sequence, rhythm, and pitch of the spoken words.

THINKING TYPE See Jung, Carl Gustav.

THOMPSON, CLARA (1893–1958). American psychoanalyst associated with Harry Stack Sullivan and known as a cultural interpersonal psychoanalyst. She was a forerunner in the field of the psychology of women and criticized Freud for his ostensible cultural bias. Thompson enjoys wide notoriety as a great teacher of the interpersonal school of psychoanalysis.

THOUGHT DISORDER Referring to schizophrenia, where primitive thinking in the form of associational disturbances becomes immediately evident. Examples include tangential thinking, word salads, concretization, syncretistic thinking, delusional thinking, and even general incoherence. Variations include

Audible thought—an auditory hallucination in which the hallucination is one of conception and not of sensation. Also referred to as the hallucination of inner voices.

Supervalent thought—obsessional intrusive thought that is impossible for the person to erase. "I can't shake it" is a typical comment from such a person.

Thought echoing—the sensation of hearing one's own thoughts emanating from the environment—either in whispers or in unbearably high-intensity decibels.

Thought hearing—the sensation of audibly hearing one's own thoughts as well as the conviction that others, too, are hearing these thoughts. The thoughts are emanating from within the person and not from the outside.

Thought pressure—also known as "insertion of ideas" or "pressure of ideas." In the neuroses, it is equivalent to invasive thoughts or "intrusive thoughts." In schizophrenic thinking it is referred to as insertion thinking, as the subject believes that another more powerful person has the power to "insert" a thought into the subject's mind.

THOUGHT ECHOING See Thought disorder.

THYMOPATHIC Refers to affect disturbance particularly with respect to feelings of pessimism, dejection, sorrow, and depression—as in dysphoric reactions.

TIC An irresistible and sudden movement of the body equivalent to a spasm. Frequently associated with Tourette's syndrome, where the person is compelled by behavior that is biologically based; these can include voice, motor, and facial tics. Also seen in children who "pick up" certain minor tic habits from observing others who exhibit them. Because of the high index of suggestibility in children, in a figurative sense, tics can become contagious. Also occurs in adults as well, who can present transitory tics as a result of stress. Tics can develop into chronic and more involuntary permanent etchings of the person's responses. As a psychological manifestation, the tic can represent some emotional conflict—theoretically assumed to be a conflict that has generated anger, which, in turn, has been repressed. The tic, as an emotional and psychological symptom, would then be considered a symbolic representation of a thwarted wish as well as appearing as the gratified wish in perverse form—as a tic. Of course, tics that are organically based would presumably not contain this sort of psychological meaning. See Stereotyped movement disorders.

TIME AGNOSIA A dysfunction in the meaning of time in all of its vicissitudes.

TOPOGRAPHICAL THEORY Freud's conception of the topography of the psyche that includes the unconscious, the preconscious, and the conscious. See Freud, Sigmund.

TOURETTE'S DISORDER See Stereotyped movement disorders.

TRACE MEMORY See Memory, trace.

TRAILING EDGE TRANSFERENCE See Transference.

TRANSACTIONAL ANALYSIS (TA) Conceived by Eric Berne. Essentially a system of psychotherapy and a paradigm or template for interaction as it is a theory of personality, a model of communication, and a study of repetitive behavior. So-called games are played in which the individual can identify the self in any number of roles or positions such as locating where the self exists with respect to the "OK" position—as in

I'm OK, you're OK—possibility for relationship is good. However, psychoanalytically, could be reflective of a hysterical diagnosis whereby everything is always OK, signifying the operation of the defense of denial.

I'm OK, you're not OK—can imply that the possibility for relationship is highly questionable. Could correlate diagnostically to paranoid rejection phenomena.

I'm not OK, you're OK—a complaining personality, always finding fault with the self so that the partner is continually bombarded with whining behavior and pessimism. Also correlates to depressive inclinations.

I'm not OK, you're not OK—a highly critical, cynical, pessimistic, fault-finding individual who is diagnostically paranoid and depressed and essentially misanthropic.

Further, TA identifies ego states of the child, parent, and adult with respect to how one assumes one of these roles in any interaction. These include:

Parent—the "taught" concept of life, ingrained voice of authority.

Adult—the "thought" concept of life, mature, realistic part.

Child—the "felt" concept of life, when anger dominates reason; impulsive.

In TA, past and present difficulties are analyzed and script analysis is used to understand the unconscious plan of the person's life.

TRANSCENDENTAL MEDITATION (TM) Considered perhaps to be a fourth level of consciousness, the other three being wakefulness, sleep, and dreaming. TM is a hypometabolic state in which everything is slowed down and the technique of meditation is designed to reduce overall tension and anxiety and increase a feeling of well-being. Perhaps better understood as a technique to quiet anger. Popularized by the Indian teacher or guru Maharishi Mahesh Yogi.

TRANSFERENCE Unconscious projection of feelings by the patient to the analyst, or conscious direction of feelings by the analyst to the patient, both based on similarity to past family figures of the person's life. Contrasts to countertransference, which is psychoanalytically defined as solely related to the analyst's unconscious transference to the patient. There are several usages of transference:

1. *Alter ego transference*—a Kohutian concept of a connection of kindredness between patient and analyst;
2. *Forward edge transference*—the reclaiming of the health of the childhood self that had been developmentally arrested;
3. *Merger transference*—a Kohutian concept of identification with the selfobject to include the analyst;
4. *Trailing edge transference*—repetition of childhood memories in the sense of acting out.

A sample of contributors to the understanding of transference and countertransference include Akhtar, Epstein, Gedo, Giovacchini, Greenson, Lasch, R. Marshall, S. Marshall, Racker, Sandler, Searles, Spotnitz, and Wolstein.

TRANSFERENCE CURE Referred to in psychoanalytic treatment as a flight into health based on the positive, optimistic, trusting, and even magical feelings the patient has for the analyst. See Flight into health.

TRANSFERENCE INTERPRETATION So-called on target interpretations regarding the patient's reactions to the therapist and the therapist's interpretation of such reactions.

TRANSFERENCE NEUROSIS Occurring within the psychoanalytic treatment process when the analyst begins to represent a nuclear family figure toward whom the patient responds by projecting affect as though the therapist were a replacement historical figure. The treatment is then to work through the conflict, as it were, on target (patient to analyst), which in psychoanalysis is considered the ultimate therapeutic aim. According to Freud, in transference neurosis, libido is directed to external instinctual objects as opposed to narcissistic neurosis, in which libido is absorbed by the ego.

TRANSFERENCE RESISTANCE Reactions by the patient to the therapist that create a conflict that serves to retard the progress of therapy. At first, the resistance can be a libidinous transference, one involving a positive attachment, but usually such resistance generates a negative transference. If this negative transference is not analyzed properly, the probability of the cessation of treatment is increased. As is the case with all resistance, repression is supported and, correspondingly, the remembering and meaningfully transformative exploration of the past is avoided.

TRANSIENT SYMPTOMS Symptoms that appear intermittently.

TRANSITIONAL OBJECT See Winnicott, D. W.

TRANSMUTING INTERNALIZATION Kohut's idea of the appearance of new self structure in the personality as a result of the optimal nontraumatic pressure of the treatment, whereby a new selfobject is acquired by the patient. In the field of neuropsychoanalysis, Watt calls affective procedural memory the core of personality, and this is considered equivalent to Kohut's transmuting internalization.

TRANSPERSONAL PSYCHOLOGY The concern of this sort of psychology includes such supranormal interests as peak experiences, mystical preoccupations, the search for the experience of bliss, as well as the search for the meaning of existence. Clinically and diagnostically perhaps a way to spiritualize one's hysteria. Yet this sort of valuation or even criticism could be made of all therapeutic modalities and theories. Jung first used the term *transpersonal* in reference to a transpersonal unconscious, which became a synonym for the collective unconscious.

TRANSSEXUALISM The experience a person has of suffering with the feeling (as well as the belief) of being in the wrong biologically gendered body. Such individuals yearn for corrective measures.

TRANSVESTITISM The need to dress in attire of the opposite sex. Most frequently seen in men. Also called cross-dressing. Noted for creating a sense of well-being and heightened sexuality in the subject.

TRAVERSAL OF FANTASY A Lacanian idea referring to a cure that reflects the aim of the analysis, that is, an analytic cure. It is what Lacan called a final struggle with the "identification with the symptom."

TRICHOTILLOMANIA See Hair pulling.

TRISKAIDEKAPHOBIA Fear of the number thirteen, especially if it falls on a Friday. It may be traced to Hangman's Day in old England, which would always be observed on a Friday. Another way to understand the superstition with Friday the thirteenth is to associate the entire obsessional problem to an unconscious antisemitic sentiment. Friday is the Jewish Sabbath eve, and thirteen is the bar/bat mitzvah year. The unconscious message of its bad luck may have insinuated Friday the thirteenth into the overall dispersion of myth, so that even Jews, not understanding its ostensible anti-Jewish message, also become triskaidekaphobic.

TRUE SELF See Self, true.

TUMESCENCE, PENILE Erection of penis.

TWILIGHT STATE A state whereby the subject can perform any number of actions without conscious awareness.

Associated with delirium states and with dissociative identity disordered persons.

TWINSHIP See Selfobject functions.

TYPE A PERSONALITY Not a psychiatric reference, but popularized to mean a hard-driving person who can also be irritable, impatient, competitive, and aggressive. Such a person is also thought to be highly ambitious and opportunistic and is usually referred to as a workaholic.

TYPE B PERSONALITY Relaxed and easygoing person who is patient and noncompetitive and seeks social interaction.

TYPOLOGY In the psychological sciences, conceiving typologies has been a tradition within personality trait theory. It is the characterization of aggregates of traits or body features that constitute an organizing principle ostensibly revealing the personality type.

U

UAO (Upper Airway Obstruction) See SAHS-UAO. See Sleep apnea.

ULTRAMARGINAL ZONE See Zone, erogenous.

UNCANNY EMOTIONS See Not-me.

UNCONDITIONED RESPONSE The original reflexive response to a stimulus that serves as the basis for establishing the *conditioned* response (pairing a new stimulus with the old one, as in Pavlov's dog). See Conditioned response.

UNCONSCIOUS (Ucs) Absence of consciousness, conscious ego, or awareness of feelings. A place where primary process material exists in a timelessness and external reality is replaced by psychic reality. Hence thoughts, although repressed, may still impact the person. Originally, the unconscious was related to the id and consciousness to the ego. However, what became clear was that ego as well as superego matter could also be unconscious. The unconscious can contain ideas, wishes, impulses, memories, and emotion. In Freud's topographic theory the unconscious is one of a tripartite system that includes

1. *the conscious*—where awareness characterizes cognition;
2. *the preconscious*—where, although material is outside awareness, it is essentially suppressed or more easily accessed;
3. *the unconscious*—where material is more deeply repressed and likely to be of a sexual nature, or of anger.

Regulation of the unconscious as well as mechanisms surrounding it are crucial to the psychoanalytic process. In intersubjective theory the unconscious is divided into three types:

1. *the prereflective unconscious*—organizing stimuli outside of awareness that influences the person's experience;
2. *the dynamic unconscious*—emotional experiences that were not expressed because they were threatening;
3. *the unvalidated unconscious*—emotional experiences that remain unexpressed because of the absence of validation from caregivers.

Lacan considers the unconscious from the point of view of linguistic laws. In the domain of neuropsychoanalytic research, the dynamic unconscious has been found to crystallize at about one and a half years of age. At this point the infant can manage two sets of feelings simultaneously:

1. *inner feelings*—feelings that are held privately;
2. *display feelings*—feelings reserved for public display.

According to Schore, the right brain "implicit self" is the psychobiological substrate of the unconscious. This right "system" is dominant for regulation of affect, stress, empathy, self-awareness, and intersubjective states. Further, according to Schore, the unconscious includes adaptive bodily based (right brain) survival functions that are not necessarily repressed, but operate too rapidly to be registered by the conscious mind (left brain). Thus the modern neuropsychoanalytic view suggests a "nonrepressed" unconscious. This also disputes the older idea that unconscious material is only sexual or aggressive. Thus any affect or motivational state can be unconscious. Analogous to Bollas's "unthought known." See Repression.

UNCONSCIOUS, COLLECTIVE See Collective unconscious.

UNCONSCIOUS FANTASY Consisting of repressed ideas that usually serve compensatory needs.

UNCONSCIOUS MEMORY See Memory, unconscious.

UNCONSCIOUS MOTIVATION See Motivation, unconscious.

UNCONSCIOUS PROCESS Referring mostly to defenses that operate automatically in order to manage emotion and control tension. According to Schore, in the domain of neuropsychoanalysis, relates to unconscious affect regulation and right brain functioning referring to both adaptive and defensive psychobiological mechanisms operating in a rapid, unconscious, and automatic manner.

UNDERACHIEVER Usually referred to with respect to academic performance insofar as the student performs to a significantly lesser standard than corresponds to that person's intellectual level and ability. Underlying anger toward a parent is usually suspect, although the awareness of such feeling is denied. Also refers to adults who have not nearly or significantly approximated their ability level or goals.

UNDOING One of the defense mechanisms within the obsessional syndrome. It is characterized by an ambivalence regarding the inclusion of new material in the subject's life. In the undoing process the person searches for symmetry in the obsessional attempt to erase some proactive behavior—that is, doing and then undoing. Also equally seen in paranoid blame psychology in which the criticality trait of the paranoid personality keeps anything alien to the self away from being accepted. Thus any momentary decision to introduce something new is then rejected (undone). See Defense mechanisms.

UNFORMULATED EXPERIENCE In intersubjectivity theory unformulated experience is experience as yet inaccessible to consciousness. Language interprets it and brings it into consciousness. Similar to Bollas's unthought known. Is also akin to as yet uncrystallized thought, so to speak, metamorphosing while in the intuitive state. See Bollas, Christopher.

UNIPOLAR Referring to depression. Usually considered the manic-depressive diagnosis in the absence of the manic component.

UNREALITY, FEELINGS OF See Depersonalization; Derealization.

UNSTRUCTURED INTERVIEW Allowing the patient an open-ended interview to permit more spontaneous expressive behavior that, in turn, allows the interviewer the opportunity to clinically assess the patient with respect to interpretive projections as well as to a sequence analysis of the patient's stream of consciousness.

UNTHOUGHT KNOWN Formulated by Bollas. See Bollas, Christopher; Intersubjectivity theory; Unformulated experience.

V

VAGINISMUS In the female, this is an inhibition of sexual functioning characterized by muscle constriction of the vagina that makes it virtually impossible for the penis to enter. Clinically considered to be a psychological-emotional symptom that is subject to cure. Etiology is thought to relate to a problem with the father. Either the father was an overpowering authority figure or a critical agency within the family or was somehow sexually threatening—whether real or imagined. Revulsion at the sexual act can also be present, or the person with such a problem may actually be interested in the sexual excitation but ultimately unable to perform.

VAMPIRISM Belief in vampires that have powers to draw blood and then affect one's presumed spiritual existence. Psychoanalytically, understood as the presence of unconsciously repressed hostility that is projected onto the world. Other theoretical precepts to explain such a belief concern oedipal as well as castration anxiety implications.

VEGETATIVE SYMPTOMS Referring to mood disorders as, for example, any major depressive disorder in which sleep, appetite, and energy level is affected.

VERTIGO Dizziness. Usually associated with acrophobia. Includes sensation of moving, spinning, or fear of falling. Can be a result of a neurological disorder or of the presence of emotional stress and conflict.

VICISSITUDES Meaning variations on a theme or the various effects and processes of a particular phenomenon. Its use in psychoanalytic works has been popularized by Freud.

VINELAND ADAPTIVE BEHAVIOR SCALES Assessing daily living skills, socialization, and motor skills from birth to ninety years. Disabilities such as dementia, autism, and a host of developmental problems are also assessed.

VISCEROTONIA Sheldon's personality type associated with an endomorphic physique. A person who loves comfort. See Sheldon, William Herbert.

VOLITION On one's own steam. Refers to the person's motivation and will.

VOYEUR OR VOYEURISM Peeping Tom whose purpose is to gain sexual gratification from spying on another. In *DSM* nomenclature, considered a paraphilia within the psychosexual disorders. Usually accompanied by masturbation and most frequently seen in men. Understood as an attempt to feel control over the object.

VYGOTSKY, LEV SEMENOVICH (1896–1934). Russian psychologist who formulated a sociocultural understanding of cognitive development emphasizing the child's inborn capacity to interact with symbols—as in written language—in contrast with Piaget, who felt that cognitive qualities evolve naturally—ontogenetically.

WAIS (WECHSLER ADULT INTELLIGENCE SCALE) The most widely used intelligence test with respect to psychological test batteries. Used clinically along with projective tests to comprise the complete psychological test battery. Contains subtests for verbal as well as for performance items and yields verbal, performance, and full-scale (combined) IQs:

Verbal Subtests

information—involves the ability to store, recall, and utilize verbal facts;

digit span—based on rote memory recall of elements in a current situation;

vocabulary—highly correlated to overall intelligence;

arithmetic—ability to focus one's concentration, revealing problem-solving facility;

comprehension—ability to utilize practical judgment and commonsense reasoning;

similarities—ability to form concepts and think abstractly.

Performance Subtests

picture completion—ability to focus on details in order to differentiate between essential and nonessential aspects of a situation;

picture arrangement—requires knowledge of interpersonal relating along with skills of planning, judgment, and perceptual organization;

block design—requires capacity for abstraction and concept formation, along with planning, judgment, visual analysis, and visual-motor coordination skills;

object assembly—involves capacity for visual-motor coordination following visual analysis and development of overall conceptualization of objects cued by their constituent parts; facility with spatial relationships is also important;

digit symbol—ability to efficiently learn new material requiring attention and concentration in a context of speed with visual-motor coordination.

See Wechsler, David.

WANDERING Used clinically as a term associated with fugue or confusional states.

WANDERLUST The need to roam rather randomly in the absence of any particular destination. Psychoanalytically, thought to imply the search for the oedipal figure and, ultimately, oedipal gratification.

WAR NEUROSIS Originally associated with shell shock, and also referred to as a traumatic neurosis, that is, a disturbance based upon a traumatic event—either physical or psychological/emotional.

WATSON, JOHN BROADUS (1878–1958). American psychologist best known as the father of behaviorism—the study of observable measurable behavior based on the scientific method. The main application of his approach was in regard to learned behavior and Pavlovian conditioning, which he introduced to American psychology. Because he posited that mental events are subjective and therefore not scientifically measurable, he has had little or no influence on the field of behavior therapy, which is based on the postulates of Clark Hull. Watson proposed that there are three basic emotions in children (fear, rage, and love), and that these are subject to conditioning. His famous study of "Little Albert" was an attempt to demonstrate the conditioning of fear in an eleven-month-old boy by presenting the child with a rat along with a loud noise. In 1913 he published his classic work, *Psychology as the Behaviorist Views It.* This work became known as the behaviorist manifesto. See Behaviorism.

WAXY FLEXIBILITY See Catalepsy; Catatonia; Schizophrenia.

WECHSLER, DAVID (1896–1981). European-born influential American psychologist who developed the Wechsler intelligence tests—the most widely utilized intelligence scales. See WAIS (Wechsler Adult Intelligence Scale).

WERTHEIMER, MAX (1880–1943). European psychologist who, along with Kurt Koffka and Wofgang Kohler, is credited as a founder of Gestalt therapy.

WET DREAM See Seminal emission.

WHITAKER, CARL (1912–1995). Important family theorist and practitioner. Saw the family as a cohesive unit rather than as discrete individuals and thus treated the family as a whole. Developed the idea of the I-ness of the infant and of the we-ness of the family. Whitaker was known as more of a forceful presence in the family therapy situation. See Family therapy.

WHITE, WILLIAM ALANSON (1870–1937). Influential American psychiatrist (neurologist and alienist) who promoted the field of psychoanalysis. The prestigious William Alanson White Psychoanalytic Institute was named for him.

WHOLE OBJECT A mature stance with respect to relationship: seeing the other person as a separate entity that needs to be treated with full rights.

WILL THERAPY See Rank, Otto

WILLIAM ALANSON WHITE INSTITUTE See Fromm, Erich.

WINNER This is one script or myth in the modality called transactional analysis where, as a result of a wish or myth of childhood, the child depicts itself in one of several possible roles. This role is then played out in the here and now in a way that corresponds to the myth and the wish.

WINNICOTT, D. W. (1896–1971). Influential British pediatrician and psychoanalyst. A theoretician who combined Freudian and Kleinian concepts within the context of his focus on the self and its relation to the mother, Winnicott saw the challenge of development as one in which healthy separation is essential, but without relinquishing ties to others. Winnicott postulated principles that either lead to normal or to psychopathological development. Attributed most psychopathology to conformity required of the infant so that natural creative play impulses were distorted into symptoms.

Annihilation anxiety—resulting from a dysfunctional condition in which the mother may not be able to meet the child's needs as well as interfering in the child's quiet time. Both conditions can cause trauma and tension. Applied to a person who experiences frequent threats to the personality because of a "thin ego" and who feels threatened by any number of interpersonal events such as intimacy, interpersonal collision, or abandonment.

Fear of breakdown—Winnicott contends that this fear, expressed in various forms of an illness syndrome, is the fear of the failure of the defense organization. This defense organization had been established against any early breakdown of the ego structure (that had already been experienced). Thus the original breakdown involved the "primitive agonies" the immature ego could not master.

Good enough mother—this is the mother who provides a reasonably responsive environment for the child. It is this good mother who provides what is necessary to create a well-fashioned holding environment that satisfies the infant's needs. The environmental provision of the good enough mother is central in the healthy development of the self and early object relations.

Holding environment—at first, in the child's development, the mother needs to create a safe, warm, loving environment—a secure one—so that the child can experience need satisfaction. Thus the important variable is what the mother provides rather than the child's instinctual pressure. In Winnicott's infant development model, this is the loving care during the phase of absolute dependence. It facilitates ego integration and ego relatedness. Ego support continues to be a need in later developmental phases. Winnicott has referred to the holding environment of the therapeutic setting.

Object usage—from the time between the child's omnipotent period and the shift to objective reality, the object (mother) is used in a completely exploitative manner. In this total appropriation of the object, it is as though the object was destroyed (used up). However, since the child can experience that the mother indeed survived (despite her sacrificial stance), a semblance and structure of the objective external world can begin to form normally.

Omnipotence—the maternal function of presenting a consistent attunement to the child is what allows the infant the illusion of omnipotence over a brief period. The mother meets the infant's needs and gestures rather than substituting her own. The infant has "created" what is there and needed. Winnicott regards this illusion of omnipotence as the basis of health, whereby life is lived creatively. See Omnipotence.

Preself disorders—psychotic, schizoid, and borderline—rely on the false self, which then devolves into psychosis, depressive disorders consisting of affective disturbances, and whole person disorders that refers to neurosis.

Squiggle game—A brief therapeutic consultation method used by Winnicott with children. It is a paper drawing interactive game. A line is drawn on a page for the child to add to. It continues as both therapist and child contribute to the drawing and the situation.

Transitional object—this is the external object that the infant adopts as the bridge in the transition from absolute dependence to relative dependence, seeing the objective reality of the mother as separate from the self. It represents the soothing aspect of the mother when she is unavailable and promotes the child's developing autonomy. It is being created by the infant, thereby belonging to him and becoming his first possession. Thus it represents the child's incremental steps of safety in the developmental process, which leads to greater autonomy and maturity.

True and false self—Winnicott conceptualized the true self and the "inherited potential" of sensory motor aliveness, which continues to be expressed and evolves with the responsive environment. The basis of the false self is the infant's reactive compliance to the mother's actions and needs. Where the true self feels real and alive, the false self experiences a lack of meaning and futility. A function of the false self is to hide and protect the true self. This split exists in every individual with a range of the degree of a false self organization. At the healthy end of the spectrum the false self is represented by the polite social self.

WISC (WECHSLER INTELLIGENCE SCALE FOR CHILDREN)

This is a frequently used intelligence test for children, ages six to sixteen years, eleven months. It contains scores on subtests for both verbal and performance items and is also utilized in the complete psychological test battery along with projective tests. Designed by David Wechsler. See WAIS (Wechsler Adult Intelligence Scale).

WISE OLD MAN In Jung's analytical psychology, the archetype of the Wise Old Man is a reference to authority and power.

WISH In the clinical applied work of psychoanalysis, the wish, although associated with impulse and striving, is more fundamentally the pleasure principle's most derivative representative in everyday life. The thwarting of the wish is, therefore, inextricably implicated in the formation of psychological symptoms. It is in the thwarting of the wish that people become angry so that as an emotion, anger, becomes arguably the most frequently experienced of all emotions, and therefore it is anger that needs to be best managed for the person to be reasonably well adjusted. When not kept conscious, but rather repressed, it is repressed anger toward the person who thwarted the wish that creates the genesis of the psychological symptom, insofar as the presence of the symptom comes to represent the gratified wish, albeit in perverse or neurotic form. See Symptom.

WISHES, FUNDAMENTAL Basic wishes are for the most part a function of compensatory needs. These are composed of wishes for recognition, security, new experience, and the hope of continuous reassuring responses from others.

WIT A function of the pleasure principle, but in a more clinical sense Freud also examined wit with reference to its possible relation to either lewd or hostile cravings that belie the person's voyeuristic or aggressive underpinnings. Thus, the tendency toward wit can be seen obliquely as a symptom, although it is also considered to be socially desirable.

WITHDRAWAL A retreat or inhibition with respect to external stimuli. Psychoanalytically, withdrawal reflects a more infantile level of functioning, with regression employed as the defense choice. Withdrawal is an overall retreat from interpersonal relationships. See Line, The.

WOLBERG, LEWIS R. (1906–1988). Influential American psychiatrist/psychoanalyst who promoted psychoanalytic training for psychologists and social workers. Along with his wife, Arlene Wolberg, in 1948 founded the Postgraduate Center for Mental Health, which, in the mid twentieth century, was reputed to be the largest outpatient psychoanalytic training and treatment center in the world, with more than 120,000 patient treatment hours per year. Wolberg was well known for his classic work on short-term psychotherapy and on hypnoanalysis. A sample of faculty, supervisors, and affiliates of the center's sixty-year psychoanalytic institute include Lucille Blum, Anthony Burry, Abraham I. Cohen, Helen Durkin, Maria Fleischel, James L. Fosshage, Edrita Fried, Max Geller, Henry Grayson, Emil Gutheil, Deborah Hample, Asya Kadis, Abraham Kardiner, Susan Kavaler-Adler, Henry Kellerman, Frank Lachmann, Zanvel Liff, Harold Leopold, Robert Marshall, Arnold Rachman, Bernard Reiss, Jeanne Safer, Clifford Sager, Harry Sands, Emanual K. Schwartz, Robert D. Stolorow, Stanley Teitelbaum, Alexander Wolf.

WOLFE, JANET L. (1941–). American psychologist. Luminary of the rational emotive behavior therapy movement, author and lecturer, and former long-term executive director of the Albert Ellis Institute. Member, editorial board, *Dictionary of Psychopathology.*

WOLF MAN The analysis by Freud of a male patient who reported a dream he had as a child in which several white wolves were sitting in a tree in front of his window. The dream was a nightmare in which the child woke in terror of being eaten by the wolves. Although many interpretations have been made, none have invited universal approval as to any so-called ring of truth. One possible clue as to the veracity of any interpretation would be to identify the person toward whom the child ran for protection; that person could likely be the culprit—the wolf. The plural of *wolf, wolves*, would represent the impulses of the culprit—the threatening figure in the dream identified as wolves or a reflection of the subject's own repressed impulses (anger and/or sexual intent) toward the culprit. The array of symptoms in this case—constipation, conversion, phobia, obsession, and anorexia, contributed to Freud's investigation of infantile sexuality. See Symptom.

WOLPE, JOSEPH (1915–1997). South African–born American psychiatrist and behavior therapy pioneer best known for his work in formulating desensitization techniques. Author of classic texts: *Psychotherapy by Reciprocal Inhibition* and *The Practice of Behavior Therapy*. See Systematic desensitization.

WORD SALAD An aspect of cognitive disturbance seen in schizophrenia in which the person mixes phrases and ideas that have no coherence and very little or no linkage. Frequently, these mixed ideas do have meaning for the patient, but in a way that is highly idiosyncratic and reflects a pathological and solipsistic self-referential focus. Referred to also as schizophasia.

WORDS, MICROCOSM OF Referring to those individuals who invest extra magical powers in words so that an obsessional paradigm is created. Within this paradigm words with personal reference take on meaning that can shake the person with emotions of fear, anxiety, dread, and overall recoiling reactions. Such persons also fully appreciate, and are grateful to hear, words that offer comfort and relief. For such people, words represent a microcosm of the macro world, and since the macro world is ostensibly difficult for such people to manage, the macro world is reflected even in the mere evocation of words. The microcosm of words then becomes an overdetermined word universe ultimately translating into a negatively charged emotion universe.

WORKING ALLIANCE Cooperative therapeutic working relationship between patient and therapist.

WORKING OUT In psychoanalysis, working out refers to the process whereby the patient and the therapist identify the parameters of the patient's life both longitudinally as well as in the here and now. Important historical and present figures are identified, the patient's geographical history is noted, and family membership is verbally diagrammed and explained.

WORKING THROUGH In psychoanalytic therapy process, working through means unraveling conflict by working on target—that is, working with transference interpretations with the therapist as the transference figure.

Off-target work is defined as working with the patient with respect to transference interpretations toward figures in the person's life other than the therapist.

WRIST CUTTING See Cutting; Self-mutilation.

X

XANAX A popular antianxiety medication.

XENOGLOSSOPHILIA Use of odd speech in the sense of pretentious speech. Reflects a focus on fantasy and withdrawal along with a reliance on the wish for adoration that fuels this unfortunate sense of achievement persona.

XENOPHOBIA Extreme fear of strangers accompanied by hostility. Seen in human groups where affiliation needs are strong and the group is especially secretive or even elite. May also be inferred as a factor in animal groups as well—perhaps in the form of territoriality. Of course, with respect to territoriality, food supply as well as issues of dominance and sexual prerogative seem to be the more specific factors of hostility to or fear of strangers.

XENOREXIA Inedible objects are sought and then ingested. It is a psychopathological symptom that reflects enough of an idiosyncratic obsessional impulse as to render the diagnosis highly suspect of psychosis.

Y

YALOM, IRVIN (1931–). Influential American group theorist and practitioner best known for his book *The Theory and Practice of Group Psychotherapy*. He is a systematizer of the data derived from dynamic group psychotherapy.

YAWNING In a strictly psychological sense yawning is frequently produced with respect to boredom. Yet boredom can be also seen as part of the glossary of disguised terms for anger. Other terms in this anger glossary would include *upset* and *dissatisfied.* Yawning out of boredom can represent the person's sense of disempowerment with the requirement of participating (albeit usually passively) in any situation that prevents the person from exiting. Disempowerment will generate anger.

YEN SLEEP Drowsiness and sleepiness that occurs when addicts are deprived of their drugs—usually morphine or heroine.

YOGA Essentially designed to calm the personality through the use of concentration and self-control. Thus distracting objects are partialed out, which is referred to as deletion of the contents of consciousness. It is a Hindu philosophical teaching that seeks what is termed spiritual unity.

YOUNG, JEFFREY E. (1950–). American behavioral therapist and creator of schema therapy, an integrative approach in the treatment of personality disorders as well as for treatment-resistive patients. See Young Schema Questionnaire.

YOUNG SCHEMA QUESTIONNAIRE. Used in assessment in schema therapy, this 232-item questionnaire includes statements one might use to describe him or herself that helps identify which core belief systems from childhood are still operative and influencing current emotions and behavior. Especially useful with personality disorders. See Schema; Schema therapy.

Z

ZEIGARNIK EFFECT Bluma Zeigarnik, (1900–1988), Russian psychologist, discovered that incompleted tasks are remembered better than completed ones. Relevant to clinical issues of memory and trauma as well as issues of self-esteem.

ZEN THERAPY Guided by philosophy of Zen Buddhism. The individual is part of the universe and the approach is to feel at one with it all. Practices include contemplation and trust in intuition.

ZILBOORG, GREGORY (1890–1959). Russian psychoanalyst known for work in schizophrenia and criminology.

ZONE, EROGENOUS Part of the body psychically invested or cathected with libidinous energy. With respect to psychosexual development, psychoanalytic understanding of the libidinous cathexis involves the oral, anal, and genital areas.

hypnogenic zone—a particular spot on the body that, when touched, can throw the person into a hypnotic trance;
hysterogenic zone—any part of the body that, when touched, can precipitate a hysterical reaction;
primacy zone—an erotogenic area that, through a series of successive approximations, spans the psychosexual trajectory beginning in the oral stage and continuing to the anal, phallic, and genital, with respect to any of these areas;
ultramarginal zones—those zones of which the person is hardly aware.

ZONE OF PROXIMAL DEVELOPMENT Difference between what the child can accomplish in the absence of mentoring. Formulated by Vygotsky.

ZOOPHILIA A paraphilia in which the person experiences sexual excitement with respect to the touching of animals.

ZOOSADISM A paraphilia in which an animal is injured for the sake of sexual pleasure.

RESOURCES

American Psychiatric Association. *Diagnostic Criteria of DSM-IV-TR*. Washington, DC: American Psychiatric Association, 2000.

American Psychological Association. *Dictionary of Psychology*. Washington, DC: American Psychological Association, 2007.

Barker, Robert L. *The Social Work Dictionary.* Washington, DC: NASW, 2003.

Campbell, Robert J. *Psychiatric Dictionary*. 6th ed. New York: Oxford University Press, 1989.

Corsini, Raymond J. *The Dictionary of Psychology.* New York: Brunner-Routledge, 1998.

Edwards, Richard L. *Encyclopedia of Social Work.* Atlanta, GA and New York: NASW and Oxford University Press, 2007.

Greenspan, S.I., N. McWilliams, and R.S. Wallerstein, co-chairpersons, Psychodynamic Diagnostic Task Force. *Psychodynamic Diagnostic Manual.* Silver Springs, MD: Alliance of Psychoanalytic Organizations, 2006.

Moore, Burness E., and Bernard Fine, eds. *Psychoanalytic Terms and Concepts*. 3d ed. New Haven: American Psychoanalytic Association and Yale University Press, 1990.

Rycroft, Charles. *A Critical Dictionary of Psychoanalysis.* New York: Basic, 1968.

Skelton, Ross, M., ed. *The Edinburgh International Encyclopaedia of Psychoanalysis*. Edinburgh: Edinburgh University Press, 2006.

VandenBos, G. R., ed. *American Dictionary of Psychology*. Washington, DC: American Psychological Association, 2007.

Varcarolis, E. M. *Manual of Psychiatric Nursing Care Plans: Diagnoses, Clinical Tools, and Psychopharmacology.* Philadelphia: Saunders, 2003.

Videbeck, S. L. *Psychiatric Mental Health Nursing.* Philadelphia: Lippincott, Williams, and Wilkins, 2007.